TAHOE RIM TRAIL

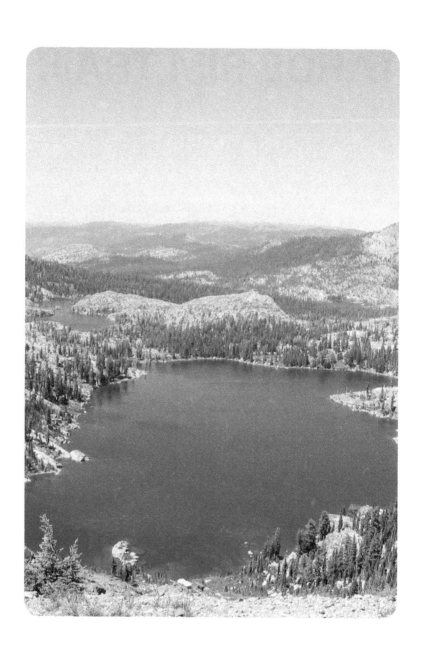

The Official Guide for Hikers, Mountain Bikers, and Equestrians

TAHOE RIM TRAIL

3rd Edition

ENDORSED BY
THE TAHOE RIM
TRAIL ASSOCIATION

Tim Hauserman

 WILDERNESS PRESS . . . *on the trail since 1967*

Tahoe Rim Trail: The Official Guide for Hikers, Mountain Bikers, and Equestrians

1st EDITION 2002
2nd EDITION 2008
3rd EDITION 2012

Front and back cover photos copyright © 2012 by the Tahoe Rim Trail Association
Interior photos, except where noted, by Tim Hauserman
Animal print illustrations by Jessica Land; illustration of "Inconsiderate Backcountry Blockhead" by Karen Schwartz
Maps: Tom Harrison, using mapping information from Jeffrey P. Schaffer
Cover design: Scott McGrew
Editor: Laura Shauger

ISBN 978-0-89997-710-2 (pbk.); ISBN 978-0-89997-711-9 (ebook);
ISBN 978-1-64359-004-2 (hardcover)

Published by: **Wilderness Press**
An imprint of AdventureKEEN
2204 First Avenue South, Suite 102
Birmingham, AL 35233
(800) 443-7227; FAX (205) 326-1012
info@wildernesspress.com
www.wildernesspress.com

Visit our website for a complete listing of our books and for ordering information.

Distributed by Publishers Group West

Frontispiece: Dicks Lake from Dicks Pass

Acknowledgments

In the fall of 2011 I raced to beat the snow to check out the 20-plus miles of new and soon-to-be-built trail, on Kingsbury Grade and above Tahoe Meadows for this latest edition. Clay Grubb and Bob Anderson, two of the incredible trail-building artists who have worked hundreds of hours to create masterpieces that we get to walk all over, joined me. A toast to all of the trail builders: Thanks for creating places for us to walk. I want to thank Mary Bennington, Jaime Souza, and Teresa Crimmins at the Tahoe Rim Trail Association for their assistance and good spirit when they heard me say, "Just one more question." Thanks to Tom Harrison for updating his maps to accommodate all that new trail.

I also want to thank all those who helped with the first two editions. In the interest of saving trees I cannot name all those who read drafts, hiked with me, gave me tips, and generally were just great to have around. But I appreciate you. I do, however, again want to thank Jessica Land and Karen Schwartz for their awesome art work. I give a bow and thank you to my editors: Jannie Dresser on the first edition which was also my first book, so you can imagine what a challenge that was, and Laura Shauger on this one, who has really helped improve my writing. I need to give special thanks to the Tahoe Rim Trail Association. Over the last twelve years the various board members and staff have always been unwavering in their assistance and support. We all have the same goal: to espouse the joys of a trail we love.

Finally I want to give kudos to my daughters Sarah and Hannah Hauserman. They graced the pages of the first edition with their little toes in Lake Aloha and are now graduating from college. Live is short—better go hiking.

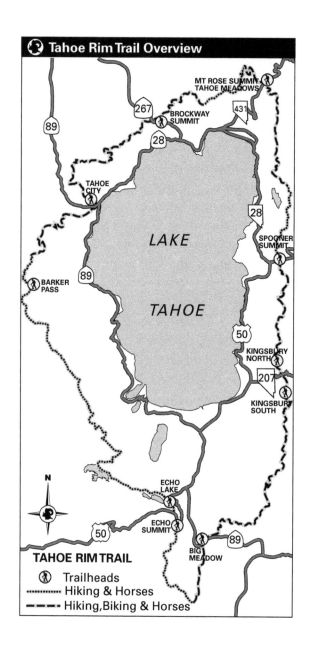

Contents

5 Fun for All and All for Fun: A User's Guide to the Tahoe Rim Trail *47*

A Hiking Paradise *47* • Backpacking and Camping *48* • Yippee! Mountain Biking *54* • Getting Horsey on the TRT *56* • Goin' Fishin' *61* • Kids Like to Hike . . . Some Kids . . . Sometimes . . . and Not Too Far *63* • What About Fido? *67*

6 Trail Description *69*

Map Legend *70*

Foreword

An organization and trail system born out of the passion and desire to create a memorable and life-changing outdoor experience, the Tahoe Rim Trail Association (TRTA) has been built on years of dedicated volunteers, staff, agency partners, and community support. In 2011 the TRTA celebrated 30 years as a nonprofit organization working hard with its partners to build and maintain *a trail like no other* . . . the Tahoe Rim Trail.

The association is grateful for support from a diverse group of outdoor enthusiasts who sustain it with tens of thousands of volunteer hours annually. Many volunteers offer their support as trail builders and maintainers, guides, ambassadors, office assistants, and board members. The TRTA's volunteer trail builders, supported by the US Forest Service and Nevada State Parks, are responsible for the layout and design of the Tahoe Rim Trail. The association's volunteers are also responsible for the trail construction and maintenance of the trail.

Thousands of workers of all ages have staked, raked, pruned, hauled, sawed, shoveled, and pried in sun and snow, dust, and rain. Many returned again and again, drawn by the camaraderie and high spirits of fellow volunteers and rewarded with a deep sense of pride in building and maintaining this magnificent public resource as their legacy. Today we continue to work with our volunteer supporters and agency partners to maintain and enhance this trail system in the Sierra Nevada.

The TRTA also inspires stewardship of this resource through guided public hikes, snowshoe hikes, outdoor skill courses, and many other opportunities to enjoy and learn about this amazing region. TRTA's segment hikes and thru-hike have become a popular way to complete the entire trail in one season with the support of the organization's trained guides and trail angels while sharing the experience with a group of fellow hikers.

Sunrise from viewpoint near Martis Peak

Tim Hauserman's guidebook serves as a wonderful tool for those interested in dayhikes, backpacking trips, mountain bike rides, runs, horseback rides, and more. We hope you will use this guide when planning your adventure in the Sierra Nevada overlooking what Mark Twain called "the Jewel of the Sierra," Lake Tahoe.

We invite you to join the famous TRTA 165 Mile Club upon completion of all eight segments of the Tahoe Rim Trail. Whether you hike it in ten days or ten years, anyone who completes the trail is welcome in this club. Upon completion of the trail, you will be asked to fill out a simple form documenting your journey. When we receive your form, we will assign you a 165 Mile Club member number and send you a certificate, pin, and patch.

The TRTA depends on the support of our many donors and members in ensuring the success of the organization. All TRTA members receive quarterly newsletters with updates on trail programs and the association, invitations to all TRTA events,

Fontanillis Lake and Dicks Peak

including the annual meeting, and an opportunity to join the 165 Mile Club. We invite you to become a member and join the family of friends who continue to support the legacy created by thousands to benefit millions for generations to come. For more information on the Tahoe Rim Trail and the association, visit **www.tahoerimtrail.org.**

Mary Bennington, Executive Director,
Tahoe Rim Trail Association, May 2012

Introduction to the Tahoe Area and the Tahoe Rim Trail

Then it seemed to me the Sierra should not be called the Nevada, or Snowy Range, but the Range of Light. And after ten years spent in the heart of it, rejoicing and wondering, bathing in its glorious floods of light, seeing the sunbursts of morning among the icy peaks, the noonday radiance on the trees and rocks and snow, the flush of the alpenglow, and a thousand dashing waterfalls with their marvelous abundance of irised spray, it still seems to be above all others the Range of Light, the most divinely beautiful of all the mountain chains I have ever seen.
—John Muir, 1912

Welcome to the Tahoe Rim Trail! This book quickly and easily provides you what you need to know to enjoy your time on this incredibly beautiful route. Having lived at Lake Tahoe most of my life, I've spent countless hours on area trails. While I am not a biologist, a geologist, a naturalist, or an -ist of any kind, I have learned enough about Tahoe plants, animals, and mountains to deepen my interest when I am in the woods. I'd like to help make your outdoor experience just as fun and fascinating.

An enormous, deep blue, subalpine lake surrounded by lofty, snowcapped peaks. Lush, green forests, dark volcanic peaks, stark granite faces, and hundreds of small, jewel-like lakes adorning the wilderness areas above this special lake. Does a place like that deserve a loop trail? Absolutely! Lake Tahoe might be the best place in the world to build a loop trail. In fact, it is quite remarkable that the trail was completed as recently as September 2001. The now 170-mile Tahoe Rim Trail (or TRT, as it is sometimes abbreviated here) circles one of the world's most beautiful lakes and winds through two states, several wilderness areas, national forest and state park lands, and an incredible diversity of geology, flora, and fauna. The trail accesses both the Sierra Nevada and its Carson Range spur, each with a unique personality. It winds through aspen meadows, skirts high mountain peaks, and runs for miles along ridgetops with stunning views. You can walk for miles under a forested canopy or saunter through meadows. You can venture above treeline for long stretches. That the trail is a big loop, a circle, may be its best feature. Wherever you set off, as the days and weeks go by, you can follow the circle back to where you began. Across the big, blue expanse of the lake, you can pick out where you were a week ago, and where you will be again in another week. Much of the multiuse Tahoe Rim Trail was constructed for the pleasure of hikers, equestrians, and mountain bikers, using modern trail-building techniques, with the goal of keeping the grade below an average of 10 percent.

Geographic Setting

Lake Tahoe is the largest subalpine lake in North America. At 22 miles long and 12 miles wide, it is a beautiful expanse of deep, blue water. What makes it so intensely blue? Its depth. At its deepest point Lake Tahoe plunges to 1645 feet with an average depth of approximately 900 feet. With its huge surface area, that's a lot of water. Tahoe is blue also because it is so clear and clean. Its clarity is primarily because the basin around it is fairly small and the water is very cold and the soils and vegetation have prevented nutrients from entering the lake where they would increase algae growth.

Since the 1960s and 1970s there has been dramatic population growth and increased development in the Tahoe area, which has had a negative effect on the lake. An increase in algae growth has reduced Tahoe's legendary clarity. A substantial investment of energy and money is now underway to protect the lake. For more information on how you can help, contact the League to Save Lake Tahoe at (530) 541-5388 or the Tahoe Regional Planning Agency at (775) 588-4547. Call or write your congressional representative and senator to ask for their support for cleaning up and protecting this lake and its surroundings. Also consult the handy list "Ways to Save Lake Tahoe" in Appendix D (page 219).

Trail History

During the 1970s when Glenn Hampton was a recreation officer for the Lake Tahoe Basin Management Unit of the U.S. Forest Service, he first had the idea of completing a trail with volunteer labor around the rim of Lake Tahoe. He forged a partnership between the Forest Service, the Nevada State Parks, and a newly created, nonprofit volunteer organization called the Tahoe Rim Trail Fund. The purpose of the partnership was to plan, construct, and maintain a Tahoe Rim Trail. Since 1984 more than 120 miles of trail have been built or improved around the lake. The Tahoe Rim Trail also uses the existing Pacific Crest Trail in the section that overlaps from Meiss Meadows to Twin Peaks.

The Tahoe Rim Trail Fund (now known as the Tahoe Rim Trail Association) is administered by a volunteer board of directors and has a small professional staff. The trail has been built partially by professional crews hired by the Forest Service or Nevada State Parks and partially by volunteers who have contributed thousands of hours. For many it has been a labor of love. Construction of the trail began in July 1984 from Grass Lake, on the north side of Highway 89 near Luther Pass, toward Kingsbury Grade. In 1985 two additional construction projects began at Spooner Summit and Tahoe City. In 2001 the last section of the trail was completed, between Rose Knob Peak and Mount Baldy.

Since that time, sections of the trail have been removed from roads and replaced with single-track trail, loops have been added, and much of the trail has been improved. In fact, with the addition of 20 new miles of trail in the last few years, which are

Tahoe Rim Trail Association

Hikers in Desolation Wilderness

included in this third edition, all of the major sections of trail that were on roads have been replaced, and several incredibly beautiful new loops have been created.

In 1999 then First Lady Hillary Rodham Clinton and the White House Millennium Council designated the Tahoe Rim Trail as the Millennium Trail for the State of Nevada. The Tahoe Rim Trail is certainly worthy of this honor, which is bestowed upon only one trail in each state, and it is destined to become one of the most popular trails in the United States, taking its place beside the Appalachian, Pacific Crest, and John Muir Trails.

The Tahoe Rim Trail Association

The mission of the TRTA is to maintain and enhance the Tahoe Rim Trail system, practice and inspire stewardship, and promote access to the beauty of the Lake Tahoe region. Funded through contributions, memberships, fundraising, grants, and the sale of merchandise, annually the Tahoe Rim Trail Association coordinates about 1,000 volunteers to work more than 10,000 hours on the trail. Over the past 30 years, the TRTA and their government partners not only built and improved the trail, but they have also built three major trailhead facilities, and a 1.3-mile wheelchair-accessible interpretive trail. The TRTA is the prime source of information for people interested in hiking, biking, or horseback riding on the Tahoe Rim Trail.

The TRTA also administers the Tahoe Rim Trail 165 Mile Club. Those who hike, ride their horses, or bike (where allowed) the entire trail can become members of the Tahoe Rim Trail 165 Mile Club.

Even though the Tahoe Rim Trail was completed in 2001, there is still much to do in order to maintain and improve the trail. Tasks include repairing damaged sections of the trail and making changes to the trail to prevent future damage. Volunteers continue to add switchbacks, change routes, add connecting trails, and do whatever is necessary to improve the trail. The newest sections of the trail can be found near the Mt. Rose and Kingsbury Grade Trailheads.

The Tahoe Rim Trail Association is key to the future of the trail and anyone can become a member. Members receive quarterly newsletters, an invitation to the annual meeting; discounts on merchandise; and the opportunity to attend TRTA-led hikes, trainings, and events—not to mention the satisfaction of knowing that you are doing your part for this wonderful trail. For more information contact the Tahoe Rim Trail Association at DWR Community Non-Profit Center, 948 Incline Way, Incline Village, NV 89451; (775) 298-0012; info@tahoerimtrail.org. Or visit **www.tahoerimtrail.org.**

Regulations and Permits

The Tahoe Rim Trail travels through three wilderness areas, which are managed by national forests: Mt. Rose Wilderness, Desolation Wilderness, and Granite Chief Wilderness. Much of the rest of the trail is on national forest lands in California and Nevada. The remainder of the trail lies in the Lake Tahoe Nevada State Park.

The only areas with limitations on hiking or camping on the TRT are Desolation Wilderness and Lake Tahoe Nevada State Park. These two include the following trail sections, described in greater detail in chapter 6.

Section 3: Mount Rose Trailhead to Spooner Summit

This section travels through Lake Tahoe Nevada State Park where camping is limited to two primitive but developed campgrounds that have picnic tables and pit toilets. A hand-operated well providing drinking water was installed at the Marlette Campground in 2010. Permits are *not* required here. For more information contact the Lake Tahoe Nevada State Park at (775) 831-0494 or the Tahoe Rim Trail Association office at (775) 298-0012.

Section 7: Echo Summit and Echo Lakes to Barker Pass

This section travels through Desolation Wilderness. Permits that can be obtained at the trailhead are required to enter Desolation Wilderness. If you are staying overnight, you must get a camping permit at the Tahoe Basin National Forest Information Center at Taylor Creek located on Highway 89 about 0.5 mile northwest of Camp Richardson. The wilderness has been divided into zones for the issuance of permits. A limited number of camping permits are available for each zone, so you may not be able to obtain a permit for the more popular areas (which tend to be lakes close to trailheads) in the middle of the summer, particularly on weekends. For more information contact the Forest Service at: Lake Tahoe Basin Management Unit, 35 College Drive, South Lake Tahoe, CA 96150 or (530) 543-2600. Or visit **www.fs.fed.us/r5/ltbmu.**

Animals and Plants, Great and Small

The Lake Tahoe area has a tremendous variety of interesting flora and fauna. You will enhance your enjoyment and experience of this beautiful region by getting to know some of them. This chapter gives a quick summary of what you may encounter as you journey along the Tahoe Rim Trail.

While many of these animals are a rare treat to encounter, the smaller animals such as squirrels and birds are found in abundance. Among the highlights of traveling in the Tahoe woods are the fascinating trees and wildflowers that you pass along the way. This book provides a quick, easily understood introduction to the most common animals and plants in the Tahoe Basin area; it is not intended to substitute for a good field guide.

The Largest Animals in the Tahoe Region

Black Bear   The largest omnivores in the Sierra are black bears, but often their fur is cinnamon brown, dark brown, reddish, and sometimes even off-white. Bears are common on the west shore of the lake, where numerous garbage cans provide a tempting place to scavenge a free meal on garbage collection days. Whether you live in the Tahoe area or are just visiting, you can do your part to protect bears—and yourself—by keeping your garbage away from where they can get to it. If you are camping or backpacking in bear country, follow these simple rules:

- Don't leave any food or clothes that smell like food in your tent. When they come to get it, you don't want to be sleeping in the path of a hungry and determined bear.

- Put your food (all your food!) in a safe place at night and when you are not in camp. If a campground has a bear-proof container use it. In the backcountry you are not only advised to put your food in a bearproof canister, but in some areas, including several wilderness areas in the central and southern Sierra, you are required to do so. The next two best methods are to hang your food high in a tree, suspended from a rope, or to put it on a 15-foot-high rocky ledge where bears can't reach it.

- Keep a clean camp so that bears or other animals won't be attracted to the site. Put food, cleaning, and fragrant hygiene supplies such as shampoo, toothpaste, and soap away soon after you are done with them.

- If you see a bear, make lots of noise. Bang pots and pans together, stand up and shout, and throw your arms around to scare it away. (Note that this approach doesn't always work!)

- Be smart. If a bear is chomping down on your food, it has already won, so don't try to take the food away from it.

- Never get between a mother bear and her cub.

- If you startle a bear, make eye contact, but do not stare at it. Instead, slowly back away and wait for the bear to amble off. Be sure not to block its escape route.

- Don't forget that bears are good runners and can climb trees.

- Treat bears with respect. Remember that you are in their territory.

While it is important to be cautious, bear attacks are extremely rare. In those very unusual circumstances where black bears have injured people, it was usually the result of human error. Be careful and enjoy them from a safe distance.

Deer The most common deer in the Sierra are named "mule deer" for their large, floppy ears that resemble those of a mule. Mule deer also sport a small white bob of a tail. Deep snow and lack of forage keep them away from the area during winter months. At that time, you are more likely to find them in the warmer climes of the Carson Valley, a short jaunt over the Carson Range from the east shore. As the season warms up, these animals are commonly spotted on the east slopes and in other areas of the Tahoe Basin.

Mountain Lion or Cougar The rare and elusive mountain lion or cougar has been seen occasionally in the Tahoe area, especially in lower elevation open areas such as the east shore and around Truckee. While I have not personally seen one on the TRT, I have seen tracks, which were following close behind a set of deer tracks. These large cats range in size from 6.5 to 8 feet long, including their tail, and can weigh up to 200 pounds. Each animal has a vast range and can cover many miles of territory in one night. Mountain lions hunt deer primarily, although they also prey on raccoons, birds, mice, and even skunks and porcupines. Porcupine?! That would have to be one hungry mountain lion.

Someone once brought a pet mountain lion to my office; its power and grace were awe-inspiring. We had the feeling that it could dispose of any one of us in half a minute. Mountain lions can jump 12 feet up a tree from a standstill. If you do encounter one, experts recommend that you do not run. Instead try to look as big as possible by standing tall, opening up your jacket, and waving your arms. Once the cat perceives that you don't behave like prey, it will probably back off. Also, a mountain lion leaves the remains of a kill and returns later to eat; needless to say, it is not wise to hang around a lion kill.

Medium-Sized Animals

Bobcat You are more likely to hear the loud scream or howl of this elusive member of the cat family than to see it With an aver-

age weight of about 20 pounds in adulthood, it is a good deal larger than an average-sized domestic cat. A bobcat has a short stubby tail that is black toward the end and tipped with white. A nocturnal preda-tor, the bobcat likes to dine on squirrels and mice. Bobcats have been sighted rarely in Tahoe Meadows, above Tahoe City, and along the west shore.

Bobcat

Coyote These adaptable creatures are common in the Tahoe area. While I've seen them in many locations, they seem to pre-fer woodlands and meadows. They can often be heard yipping

and howling at night in Ward and Blackwood Canyons, Squaw Valley, Alpine Meadows, and other places. Though coyotes resemble medium-sized dogs, they are much more graceful and lis-some when they run, a sight to behold. It is not uncommon for a dog to chase a single coyote, only to discover that the coyote is leading him back to

Coyote

his teammates. Although many people believe that coyotes do not hunt in packs, I have seen them several times in groups of three or four adults. If you live in the mountains, take care with your domesticated animals, even around your home. Many a lost cat or small dog has become a coyote dinner.

Marten It is a rare treat to spot a marten, also called a pine marten. At about 1.5 to 3 feet long, including its tail, the marten is about the size of a housecat but longer and sleeker. Martens have beautiful lush brown fur and long bushy tails. They are agile climbers and sometimes live in a cavity high up in a tree. They are elusive animals, but can occasionally be seen in pursuit of squirrels or chipmunks, their favorite dinner. Several years ago I saw one in nearby trees around my Tahoe area house for about two weeks. The grace and stealth of the marten is unmatched.

Marmot If you hear a high-pitched squeak when you are walking by a big rock pile, there is a good chance that it harbors a yellow-bellied marmot. Also known

Marmot

as woodchuck, the marmot is about the size of a housecat. Related to squirrels, marmots are dark brown and cinnamon in color, live in groups and love to sun themselves on rocks. I have often seen them in Desolation Wilderness, on the Pacific Crest Trail near Twin Peaks, and in the Mt. Rose area.

Porcupine These large rodents can often be seen on roads or sitting up in a tree. About 2 to 3 feet long, they are large and round with short legs. They have light brown to yellowish fur and numerous hollow but sharp quills of up to 3 inches long. The porcupine walks in a slow, lumbering fashion—if no one wants to eat you, why hurry?—and enjoys a diet of succulent bark and herbaceous plants. No animals, except cougars perhaps, want to have anything to do with these quill-covered critters, and although their quills can cause others a great deal of pain, especially to overzealous dogs, it is a myth that they can "shoot" their quills.

Raccoon These carnivorous little burglars are one of the most interesting animal species in the Sierra. Their distinctive face looks like a burglar's mask, with a black band across the eyes and a

Raccoon

mostly white face. They range in size, but can get as big as a medium-sized dog. Raccoons are nocturnal—all the better to wake you in the middle of the night while they are knocking over garbage cans in pursuit of food. It is common to see them on house decks but rare to see them in the wild. Often the best evidence of a raccoon is the very distinctive handlike tracks they leave.

Small Animals

These ubiquitous rodents inhabit the ground, the trees, perhaps even your attic, and represent a fair percentage of local roadkill. A recent squirrel census reported 178 million squirrels in the Tahoe Basin.

California Ground Squirrel   These squirrels have large bodies like the gray squirrels but have much smaller tails. They have a mottled brown coat and a silver saddle over the shoulder. They spend most of their time on the ground and are very busy all summer getting fattened up to hibernate through the winter.

Chickaree or Douglas Squirrel   This medium-sized dark brown squirrel has a reddish tinge on its back, a white belly, and a bushy tail with a silver tip. Chickarees stay active all winter and make a short explosive *quer*-o sound.

If you hear fir cones crashing down to the ground, and see the mangled remnants of the soft cones sitting on a stump, you will know you are in chickaree country. These squirrels love to climb trees and drop the cones for later, when they remove the entire cone, piece by piece, in order to get to the tasty seeds inside.

Golden-mantled Ground Squirrel and Chipmunk   What is the difference between a chipmunk and the golden-mantled ground squirrel? A chipmunk is smaller and has lines on its back that go all the way over its head. The Tahoe area's most common squirrel, the golden-mantled, has a lovely white band bordered by black running up each side of its back and ending at its shoulders. To complicate matters there are a number of different chipmunk species with minor differences in appearance. Both

Golden-mantled ground squirrel

chipmunks and ground squirrels eat seeds, grasses, and fruit.

Western Flying Squirrel These small brown squirrels (smaller than a chickaree) are very friendly and social, but since they are nocturnal most people will not have the opportunity to see one. They don't fly but rather glide through the air from tree branch to branch. Like the western gray squirrel, the flying squirrel remains active all winter.

Western Gray Squirrel Larger than either the chickaree or ground squirrel, the gray squirrel also lives in the area but in smaller numbers. It has a uniform gray body and a long, broad tail. Like the chickaree and unlike the ground squirrels and chipmunks, the gray squirrel is active all winter. It loves to sit in trees and "laugh" at cats and dogs, which stare at it with evil intent.

Pika or ***Cony*** The pika is smaller than a chipmunk, light brown in color, and lives primarily in high rocky areas. It looks like a cross between a chipmunk and a small rabbit (and is in the same animal order as the latter) with shorter ears. It makes a peeping noise.

Birds

American Robin Slightly smaller than the Steller's jay, the robin has a similar physique and is a frequent summer visitor to Lake Tahoe. With its brick-red breast, yellow bill, and gray back, the robin cheerily hops through the understory of local woods or meadows, looking for insects or worms.

Bald Eagle   A very large, majestic black bird with white head, the bald eagle occasionally is spotted flying near water, perched on a large tree, or riding the updrafts. I remember watching an eagle fly along the lakeshore, when suddenly two ospreys began to chase it; the three completed some incredible acrobatic stunts before the ospreys gave up. Perhaps the eagle had ventured too near the osprey nest. Count yourself lucky if you see one of these rarer raptors.

Blue Grouse   You are more likely to hear a blue grouse than to see one. Males vocalize a very low, bass-drum brrrmmmmmmm, br-rrmmmmmm, brrrmmmmmm sound. Females are large, plump birds about the size of a pheasant or chicken. Their plumage is brownish gray with some white feathers near their neck. They can sometimes be seen in trees or brush. Breaking cover, they startle you as they suddenly take flight with a loud wap, wap, wap of wings. This bird can commonly be seen or heard in heavily wooded sections on the west shore, including Desolation Wilderness and areas north of Tahoe City.

Canada Goose   Commonly seen along Tahoe beaches and in parks, this large grayish-tan goose has a black head and neck and a prominent white chin. Though geese are known to steal food from unsuspecting small children, they are beautiful when flying in their A-line formations. Less beautiful are the copious amounts of droppings they leave, making a trip to many a Tahoe beach akin to walking through the room of a teenager (messy but not dangerous). Similar to the Canada geese, but rarer are snow geese, which occasionally can be seen flying in large groups above the Sierra. It is a site to behold, but you will hear their raucous cries long before you see them.

Clark's Nutcracker   With a shape and sound similar to the Steller's jay, this light gray bird has black wings with white patches. Seen at treeline along high ridgetops, very much Tahoe Rim Trail country, Clark's nutcracker makes a loud and slow flap, flap,

flap with its wings as it flies from tree to tree. It prefers whitebark pines; a single bird can bury thousands of pine seeds in a summer season.

Mountain Bluebird   A rare and beautiful treat, the mountain bluebird is sky blue and startling in its soft beauty. About the size of a robin, it is a lighter blue than the much more common Steller's jay. Look for it in grassy meadows or at the edge of the forest hunting insects. I have seen it in Ward Canyon and near Truckee.

Mountain Chickadee   Perhaps the most common bird in the Tahoe woods, the small chickadee (about 5 inches long) is light gray with a black cap and white line over each eye. Usually quiet, this active bird may be best known for its call, which many people say sounds like cheese, burrr, gerrrr; others claim its call sounds more like tsick-a-dee-dee-dee. You be the judge. Maybe it just sounds like the voice of a chickadee.

Mountain Quail   California's state bird is small to medium-sized and slightly chunky. You can identify it by the little standard issuing from the top of its head, its gray to brown coloring, and the way it scurries away into nearby brush. It stays close to the ground under bushes near sunny open areas and water sources. Since quail convene in coveys, once you spot one, you will likely hear and see others.

Osprey   Another rare bird, the osprey is best known for its ability to swoop down and catch fish in its talons. The osprey is a little smaller than an eagle, with brown feathers on its back and white feathers on its breast. When flying above you, it appears mostly white, but while sitting in a nest with wings tucked, it can appear mostly brown. The osprey makes a high-pitched squeak and can be seen along the lakeshore or high up in large nests it has built out of sticks at the top of dead trees. I have watched an osprey dive into Dicks Lake and remove fish that were feeding in the evening.

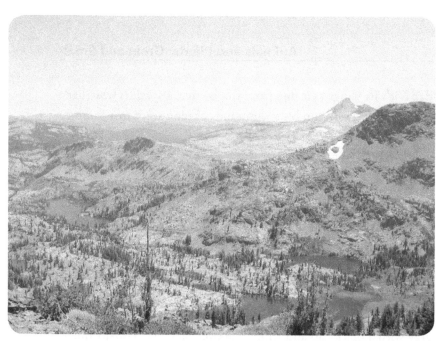

View from Dicks Pass

Owl   Various species of owl inhabit the Tahoe area. Primarily nocturnal, they live in the deep woods and are more likely to be heard than seen. While the calls of owls vary with the species, in general you can hear a deep who, who, who. Owls have large, round faces with piercing front-facing eyes perfect for late night hunting. Some species have catlike ear tufts that stick straight up.

Steller's Jay   The seemingly ubiquitous Steller's jay is most often found at lake-level elevations and in campgrounds. It is medium-sized with a dark blue body and a black mantle, throat, and crest. Its aggressive raucous cry or squawk is distinctive. It will eat your potato chips and raid your snack packs, yet many Eastern birders delight in seeing this bird for the first time.

Western Tanager   Though somewhat uncommon, the tanager is one of the most colorful birds in the Tahoe area. The male has a red head, a bright yellow body, and black wings. The female is also bright yellow but has a less dramatic greenish-yellow head. Try to spot this small to medium-sized bird (bigger than a chickadee, smaller than a Steller's jay) flitting from tree to tree.

Amphibians and Reptiles

Pacific Tree Frog   These tiny frogs can be heard in many Sierra locales. They are especially common in the grassy area around Twin Lakes, so if you're walking to these lakes be careful not to step on them. About 1 inch long, the frogs are brown or green with black eye stripes. Though called tree frogs, they have no special preference for trees and are just as comfortable on the ground or in the grass.

Snakes   Several snakes live in the Tahoe area. Happily for area hikers, the rattlesnake is not common among them. The most common snake in the Tahoe area is the garter snake. It is about 2 feet long or less and slender with a tail tapered to a sharp tip. The garter snake has a black or gray upper surface with a yellow line along its back. While for the most part it is harmless, if handled it may discharge a foul-smelling liquid. Less common to this area is the rubber boa. A wonder to behold, this docile, harmless small brown snake is usually less than 2 feet long. With its smooth skin, it looks like a worm on steroids.

Western Fence Lizard   This 6- to 9-inch lizard is often found in dry areas lounging on a rock or running to escape your big feet. The scaly skin of the lizard is gray, and they are often seen doing "push-ups" on the rocks, exposing their blue bellies.

Insects

Bees, Yellow Jackets, and Wasps   Honeybees and bumblebees quietly go about their business of pollinating flowers and rarely sting people. Yellow jackets, even though they look like a bee, are actually a form of wasp. After an above-average winter snowfall, especially in a season with a lot of spring moisture and cold temperatures, yellow jackets are found in small numbers. In drought conditions, however, yellow jackets multiply, and by late summer and fall they can be a nuisance. They are ferocious predators and carnivores, and their stings can be painful and cause swelling. These wasps can nest in the ground or in a trail-side log. If you get too close to their nests, they will come out in force to sting you. Wasps are most active from midday to just after sunset.

Mosquitoes   These pesky little critters are usually a problem from mid-June through mid-July throughout the Tahoe area. The timing of their emergence from the shadows of spring, however, depends on the quantity of precipitation that arrived during winter and how quickly the snowpack melts. Mosquitoes are active at dusk and dawn and are prevalent in shady forest areas, as well as in and near meadows, along a lakeshore, near creeks, and near any body of standing water or moist area. They especially like small, shallow bodies of water where they breed. To avoid mosquitoes, either pack a lot of insect repellent (or lemon eucalyptus), take to a granite mountain or ridgetop area, or pray for wind.

Fish

Fish have not been seen recently on the Tahoe Rim Trail, but there are some in the streams and lakes that you might pass. Here are the few to look out for:

Brook Trout   Not a true trout, but a char, its lighter colored spots on a dark green-gray background distinguish the brook. It also has a yellow- to ruddy-colored underbelly. It can be found in any Sierra water source, but is especially common in small creeks and streams.

Brown Trout   Hugging river bottoms, the brown trout sports an olive-green to cinnamon-brown coloring with reddish spots along their sides. These fish were imported into the Sierra from Germany and Scotland.

Cutthroat Trout   The most common fish in the mountain lakes and streams, the cutthroat can be identified by its red, orange, or yellow "slash" marks under each jaw. It is sometimes called the spotted trout.

Kokanee Salmon Introduced in the 1940s into the Tahoe area lakes, the kokanee can be found here still. It has a robust body and dusky olive to bluish coloring. It is silvery on its underside and nests in bottom gravel like the rainbow trout. During their fall spawning run, they turn bright red and can be found in large numbers in Taylor Creek, on Lake Tahoe's South Shore. Sometimes they are also found in smaller numbers spawning up Eagle Creek, right next to Vikingsholm Castle near Emerald Bay.

Mackinaw or Lake Trout Incorrectly blamed for eliminating the cutthroat from Lake Tahoe, the mackinaw trout is also a char family member like the brooky mentioned above. It is gray with some yellow speckles that brighten during spawning season, the least colorful of all the Sierra fish. It grows to a large size; every year 20- to 30-pound mackinaws are caught in Lake Tahoe and Donner Lake, and 10-pound fish are common.

Rainbow Trout With a bluish-gray to gray-green back, silvery belly, and dark black speckles, the rainbow's most distinctive mark is a red streak down each side. Mountain men and prospectors introduced rainbows into the Sierra in the 1800s.

Trees

Aspen or Quaking Aspen The Sierra's most colorful deciduous tree derives its name from the appearance it has when its leaves quake in gentle breezes or windstorms. With white bark and oval-shaped leaves, aspens are common in wet and moist areas, along creek beds, near springs, and in meadows. Their presence can indicate a groundwater source. Aspen trees spread by cloning themselves by means of root suckers, which grow up into more aspens around the base of their trunks; a single tree may put out dozens of shooters and thus a whole grove may have started with one tree. This tree provides most of the Sierra's fall yellow and gold color.

Cedar tree

Incense Cedar These trees can grow to a height of 150 feet. Incense cedar is commonly found near the lake (6200 feet) with an upper elevation of around 6500 feet, a little higher in sunny locations. Incense cedars have red to cinnamon-brown flaky bark, and dark green short needles, which lie in flat feathery groupings.

Jeffrey Pine Jeffrey pine is the dominant pine tree in much of the Tahoe Sierra and, though it is especially prevalent near lake level, it can grow at elevations up to 8000 feet. The Jeffrey pine can reach a height of 180 feet. It has thick gray to reddish bark, which turns redder as the tree matures, and smells like butterscotch, vanilla, or pineapple, depending on what kind of nose you have. It also has large roundish cones with upturned prickles and long needles of three.

Lodgepole Pine This usually straight tree (hence its value as a lodge pole for Native Americans) is very common in a variety of soil conditions from below 6000 feet to higher than 9000 feet in elevation. It has thin, scaly, light gray, sappy bark and small cones. The needles are in bunches of two and can be made into an "L" for lodgepole. The tree prefers wet areas, and its presence often signals mosquito territory.

Mountain Hemlock Mountain hemlock prefers high snow areas above 7000 feet and are common above 8000 feet in many north-facing areas along the Tahoe Rim Trail, generally in areas of maximum snowpack. A beautiful and majestic tree reaching heights of 25 to 100 feet, with smaller trees at the highest elevations, mountain hemlock has short, dark green needles on branches that cover the tree from bottom to top. The branches have a gentle sloping appearance; the cones are small and dark brown. What makes the mountain hemlock especially magical is the way the top of the tree droops over like a wizard's hat.

Ponderosa or Western Yellow Pine Similar to the Jeffrey, the ponderosa prefers lower elevations, usually below 6500 feet, and grows in smaller numbers near Lake Tahoe. It has yellowish to reddish-brown bark and often reaches heights of 100 feet. Like Jeffrey pine, ponderosa also has long needles of three. Ponderosa pine cone prickles stick up and out, while the Jeffrey's turn up and in (remember "gentle Jeffrey" or "prickly ponderosa"). Some areas have a hybridized combination of Jeffrey and ponderosa, making identification difficult.

Red Fir White firs' red cousin dominates the landscape in some areas above 6500 feet, often living in dense stands. The red fir needle bunches are tighter than those of the white fir, curve inward, and grow to longer than an inch. The bark is reddish-brown to gray, and the tree sprouts medium-sized cones of 6 to 9 inches as compared to the shorter ones of white fir (3 to 5 inches).

Sugar Pine These beautiful, majestic trees can reach a height of 250 feet. They are rarely seen above 6500 feet and only occasionally

Trees and Altitude

Trees in the Sierra tend to find their niche at a particular altitude. By knowing your altitude, you might be able to identify the tree; conversely if you can identify a tree, it might help you determine your altitude. The one exception to the rule is the lodgepole pine, which seems to be found at nearly any mountain elevation. The chart below details where trees are dominant. Be aware that you may find a few stragglers above and below the listed ranges. But if, for example, you see lots of western white pines and no sugar pines, you will know that you are above 7000 feet in elevation.

6000–6500 feet White fir, Jeffrey pine, ponderosa pine, sugar pine, lodgepole pine, aspen, and incense cedar

6500–7000 feet Red fir, Jeffrey pine, lodgepole pine, and aspen

7000–8000 feet Hemlock, western white pine, red fir, mountain juniper, and lodgepole pine

8000–9000 feet Hemlock, western white pine, juniper, lodgepole pine, and whitebark pine

Above 9000 feet Whitebark pine

seen in lower elevations since most were cut down for lumber at the end of the 19th century. The sugar pine has long cylindrical cones that grow 10 to 16 inches downward from the tips of long graceful branches. John Muir said of the sugar pine that it "is the noblest pine yet discovered, surpassing all others not merely in size but also in kingly beauty and majesty."

Western (Sierra) Juniper   Often junipers are found in dry, rocky areas at higher elevations—particularly in the Desolation Wilderness. Junipers more than 1,000 years old have been found in the Tahoe area. They have an appearance similar to incense cedars with reddish, brown bark. They rarely exceed 50 feet in height. Those growing in windy, exposed areas may be twisted and gnarled. The best way to tell the difference between juniper and incense cedar is that juniper has blueberrylike berries and is usually found at higher elevations. Scratch and smell one of these blue berries, and you will quickly discover that they are used to make gin.

Western White Pine   These trees grow at elevations of 7000 feet to 9000 feet and can reach 150 feet in height although they are usually much smaller because of the harsh conditions in which they live. Like the whitebark pine, the western white pine has needles that come in clusters of five. Its cone resembles that of the sugar pine though it is shorter (6 to 8 inches) and narrower. The upper branches of a western white pine, also known as silver pine, turn upward at their tips. Mature trees have a distinctive checkerboard pattern on their bark.

White Fir   Probably the most common tree in the Tahoe Basin, white fir typically grows below 6500 feet in elevation (although they are sometimes seen up to 7500 feet). They have gray bark and short, bunched needles that have an average length of 1.5 to 2 inches and a flat appearance. The bark of younger trees is somewhat smooth; as the trees age, the bark gets rougher and more like that of other pine and fir trees. The light green upright cones are soft and found scattered about the woods—the work of chickarees.

Whitebark Pine This high-elevation tree is usually found near mountaintops and is easily mistaken for a lodgepole pine. The tree has short stiff needles clustered in groups of five (while the lodgepole needles are in groups of two). The bark is gray-white, and the cones are small and dark brown. It is also common to see them near the tops of peaks in a shrublike formation called krummholz, where they may only stand a foot or so high.

Wonderful Wildflowers

Wet Areas: Meadows, Stream Banks, and Springs

Corn Lily This poisonous plant looks somewhat like a stalk of corn, but smells like cabbage. Not only is its poison deadly, but it has been reported to turn its victims green. The corn lily starts out like a big cigar popping out of the moist meadows in the

Corn lilies

spring, which by late summer grows to 3 to 6 feet tall. At the top of its broad-leaf stalk, it shows a large grouping of cream-white flowers.

Cow Parsnip A large wildflower with huge maple-shaped leaves, cow parsnip stalks can reach up to 10 feet tall but average 4 to 5 feet. It is often found in meadows, along creeks, or in other moist areas. It has several tall stalks with tight white button flowers that look like miniature cauliflower heads at the top.

Crimson Columbine The most commonly seen columbine of the Tahoe area has numerous bright red-orange flowers that look like miniature Chinese lanterns hanging off tall, thin stalks. It grows to about 3 feet high in moist meadow areas and along streambeds.

Delphinium or ***Larkspur***   Towering larkspur or larkspur delphinium have tall narrow stalks with beautiful small purple flowers that bloom all along the stalks. They are found in large numbers in some meadow and stream areas and provide a dramatic display, especially when they reach their maximum height of 6 to 8 feet. Nuttall's larkspur is a smaller variety at only about 1 foot high; it is found in limited numbers in dry or wet areas.

Elephant Heads   Sprouting off the foot-tall green stalks are numerous tiny pink flowers shaped like elephant trunks and ears. While not as showy as other meadow plants like columbine and tiger lilies, elephant heads are often seen in spring and early summer in Tahoe Meadows and especially in Meiss Meadows.

Monkeyflower   There are 11 species of this plant in the Tahoe area, all having flowers that supposedly resemble little monkey faces. The most common are the pink Lewis's monkeyflower and the yellow common monkeyflower. They favor the banks of small streams or seeps throughout the Tahoe area.

Monkshood   This relatively uncommon plant is found in moist areas. Its large deep purple flower resembles a monk's cowl. A tall plant that can reach 6 feet, monkshood grows among the tremendous variety of flowers found near Marlette Lake as well as in the Page Meadows area.

Shooting Stars   Found in moist meadow areas, shooting stars have delicate petals that bend back to expose their darker stamens, thus making them like stars streaking across the night sky. The alpine shooting star has pink flowers, while the Jeffrey's has a purple to pink flower with a black point and a small band of yellow just above the black.

Tiger lily

Tiger (Alpine) Lily   Often found with columbine in wet or marshy areas, the tiger lily can grow 4 to 6 feet tall and is a wonderful visual treat with bright orange flowers speckled with brown.

Dry and Sunny Areas

Checkermallow   Along with mules ears, this is perhaps the commonest flower in dry, volcanic areas. It is found at lake level and up to more than 9000 feet and is a low-lying flower with small pinkish-purple cups threaded by white veins.

Deep Forest Pinedrops   The pinedrop is a saprophyte, which means that the plant obtains its nutrients from decaying vegetation in the ground rather than through photosynthesis. Pinedrops grow to 4 feet tall and have orange-red to reddish-brown stalks with numerous little curlicues coming off the sides of each narrow stalk. After they die they often remain standing for years, turning darker as years go by.

Douglas or ***Sierra Wallflower***   This bright-yellow flowered plant is common in dry areas and on rocky slopes. A member of the mustard family, it has a big cluster of little yellow petals forming a ball atop a straight green stem. It reaches a height of 1 to 3 feet.

Fireweed   Fireweed grows in profusion along old road cuts and areas that were recently burned, disturbed, or where most of the plant cover has been removed. It seems to be most prolific after drier-than-normal winters. The plants are 3 to 4 feet high and covered with bright pink flowers.

Horsemint   Horsemint is found in abundance in dry meadows and on rocky flats (Tahoe Meadows is one example). It is identifiable by its purple corn-cone group of flowers situated on top of a green stem with many green leaves. It is related to pennyroyal.

Mariposa Lily   The beautiful round white flowers of the Mariposa lily have a purple to black center and a delicate appearance.

Mariposa lilies

Three cream-white petals form a small bowl. This plant is usually shorter than 6 inches and prefers dry or sandy soil on sunny open slopes.

Mountain Pennyroyal or ***Coyote Mint*** This common flower grows in open forests and along volcanic slopes. A member of the mint family, pennyroyal has white or pink flower clusters atop upright stalks. It provides a strong mint smell as you walk by.

Mules Ears In areas with open, south-facing slopes, and particularly with volcanic soils, the mules ears are often the dominant flower species. They can cover acres of land with very few other plants in view. When you see a field of mules ears, you will also smell them as they have a strong odor. Big yellow sunflowers and large leaves that resemble the ears of a mule lend the plant its name. In the fall, the leaves dry up and turn brown, and make a rustling noise in the wind.

Prettyface These relatively common flowers grow close to the ground and have 6 light yellow petals at the end of each flower stem. Each petal has a small dark purple line extending toward its tip. Large groups of "pretty faces" can be found looking at you from dry soil.

Scarlet Gilia The bright red-orange beauty of scarlet gilia is startling to behold when it appears in the dry sandy forest and on open slopes. It can get up to 3 feet tall and has many bright trumpet-shaped flowers.

Snowplant Snowplants are also saprophytes and do not require sunlight to

Snowplant

grow; they appear near trees or in dense forest areas. They are long and cylindrical (from 6 inches to 1 foot high) and a bright red color. Snowplant shoots straight out of the ground like a huge asparagus stalk, adding a splash of red color to the shade of the forest. They get their name because they pop up just after the snow melts.

Mixed Wet or Dry Areas

Asters and *Daisies* There are several species of these sunflowers that have pale purple petals circling a disk of yellow or gold. The western aster and wandering daisy are both quite common in the Tahoe area. Both plants grow up to 2 feet tall, although they are usually shorter, and occur up to 9000 feet. They prefer moist over dry settings.

Asters

Explorer's Gentian This late-season bloomer has deep blue or purple tubular-shaped flowers. Light dots speckle the inside of the petals. Found in moist or rocky terrain, gentian provides a bit of bright color when many summertime flowers have come and gone.

Lupine One of the Tahoe region's most common flowers, lupine is found in a number of different varieties. The common feature is that the leaves, no matter how small or big, are palmately shaped, which means they form groups like a hand. In the Sierra most lupines show off deep purple flowers. Tall large leaf lupines are found in abundance in wet areas, such as between Meiss Meadows and Showers Lake. Other large lupines include Torrey's and Tahoe lupine. Brewers lupine is a high-altitude low-lying lupine with tiny leaves and dark purple flowers.

Paintbrush The orange Red Applegate's paintbrush and the giant red paintbrush are the two species most commonly seen in the Tahoe area. Both have flowers that look like the brush end of a bright orange and red paintbrush. Often they are called Indian paintbrush. These and other species can be found on dry slopes to wet meadows, up to 9000 feet.

Paintbrush

Shrubs and Bushes

Buckthorn, Snowbush, or ***Mountain Whitethorn*** This plant with many names grows along disturbed areas, such as trails, and has lots of narrow white branches with spiny, thorny tips; when flattened by the snow, these branches lay down over the trail. I call it "mountain bikers' menace" because its thorns can puncture tires. Whitethorn is about 3 to 4 feet tall and spreads out over 5 to 10 feet. It has small ovate-shaped whitish or green leaves. Often the plants are so thick that it is difficult to determine where one plant ends and another begins.

Chinquapin This common plant was named after a condominium project north of Tahoe City (or was it the other way around?). Chinquapin is a bushy shrub related to oaks that inhabits dry slopes and rocky ridges and frequently grows near manzanita bushes. The narrow leaves of this 2- to 4-foot-tall plant are up to 3 inches long, yellow-green on the top, and yellow-brown underneath. Chinquapin produces yellow-green seedpods in spring.

Huckleberry Oak One of the most common plants in this area, huckleberry oak typically gets up to about 3 feet high and grows on dry south-facing slopes. It has small leathery ovate leaves of medium to dark green. At the end of the narrow stalks you may see a light green acorn.

Manzanita While there are five species of manzanita in the Sierra, only two are commonly seen in the Tahoe area. Greenleaf manzanita is widespread in dryer areas over a wide elevation range.

Its smooth bark is dark red or reddish-brown with shiny, bright green leaves, and it grows to about 3 to 5 feet tall. Manzanita has lots of rigid, crooked thick branches. In the spring they put out tiny pink flowers that supposedly look like little apples (*manzanita* is Spanish for "little apple"). Pinemat manzanita, with smaller leaves and stalks, is a smaller plant that grows to about a foot tall; it likes to form a carpet along the ground or over the top of granite rocks. Pinemat manzanita usually grows at a higher altitude than its greenleaf cousin. It is especially common between South Camp Peak and Kingsbury Grade.

Red Mountain Heather This dwarfish bush has dark green coniferlike needles and clusters of small bright pink or red flowers on the top of short stalks. It grows at high elevations throughout the Tahoe area, along some lakeshores, and in the Desolation Wilderness. This fragile plant is a thick ground cover running alongside the trail—take care not to step on it.

Squaw Carpet or ***Mahala Mat*** Thick patches of this plant as much as 10 to 20 feet across are made up of hollylike leaves carpeting the ground. In the spring, clusters of small blue to violet flowers grow among the sharp-edged leaves.

Thimbleberry They may not keep you from starving in the woods, but thimbleberries are edible and quite tasty when they ripen in late August and September. They are in the same family as blackberries and raspberries, and you will not be surprised to hear that the berries look like little thimbles. This bush is usually found in large groups lying close to the ground near streams and in other shady moist areas. Thimbleberry has large leaves that resemble a maple leaf with three to five pointed lobes. The showy white flowers bloom in early summer.

Tobacco Brush This plant is also called snowbrush ceanothus and curlleaf ceanothus. Some say the strong pungent aroma of tobacco brush is sensuous and aromatic; to me, it smells like tobacco.

Islands await at Middle Velma Lake.

With large, shiny, dark greenish-blue leaves, the plant grows up to 5 feet tall and has numerous small white flowers. Tobacco brush likes dry disturbed areas along road cuts and trails and can become the locally dominant plant.

Let's All Get Along:
A Trail for Everyone

The goal of the Tahoe Rim Trail Association is for all users to safely use and enjoy the trail while working to maintain and protect it. It is important that all trail users pleasantly coexist. Doing so comes down to understanding and being courteous to one another, and through recognizing that we are all out there to have fun. Hikers affect the Tahoe Rim Trail less than mountain bikers do. Although horse traffic has the greatest effect on the quality of the trail, there are far fewer horseback riders than other trail users. The only way to make sure that relations between the user groups improve and that the TRT is maintained is for users to follow some simple rules.

Rules for Mountain Bikers

When the Tahoe Rim Trail was first constructed, hiking and horseback riding were allowed, but mountain biking was prohibited on the entire trail. As opposition to mountain bike use declined and the numbers of riders increased, much more of the trail has been opened to bikers. Where bikes are allowed, bike riders are often the major trail users. Now you can ride a mountain bike on over half the trail.

While people both hike and ride, there can still be tension between the different types of trail users. Since mountain bikers have become major trail users and bike use continues to be controversial in some eyes, mountain bikers should make an extra effort to be

🚲 Dirt Users' Hints

Preserve the Dirt

- 🚲 Skidding destroys trails. Learn to use both brakes like the pros.
- 🚲 Stay on the trail! Deadfall trees? Snowbanks? Hurdle them—you're tough.
- 🚲 Stay in the center of the trail. Preserve a single-track trail as a single track.
- 🚲 Yes, you do need written approval from the controlling land agency to build your dream trail.
- 🚲 Join multiuse maintenance crews. Help preserve the trail's integrity.

Respect Other Users

- 🚲 Pass others at a socially acceptable velocity—for them!
- 🚲 Ring a bell, smile, and say hello.
- 🚲 Horses think you want to eat them. Act accordingly; wait on the lower side of the trail.
- 🚲 Wear a helmet, or others will have to drag your corpse back to your loved ones.
- 🚲 Ride only open trails. Remember the PCT, wilderness areas, and several other portions of the Tahoe Rim Trail are closed to bikes. You need to know if the portion of trail you want to bike on is open to bikes.
- 🚲 Leave nothing of your presence behind. That includes trash, skid trenches, and off-trail tracks.

courteous and sensitive to the environment by remaining on the maintained trails. They should urge friends and others that they meet to do so as well.

Cycling is a legitimate use of backcountry trails, but there are responsibilities that all bikers are expected to assume. Hikers have complained about encountering bikers on sections of the trail closed to biking, while many hikers, trail runners, or horseback riders have been surprised or threatened by bikers speeding past.

The Tahoe Rim Trail Association has published the Dirt Users' Hints, the rules of the trail for bikers (see sidebar).

Hikers Take Note

In recent years, mountain bikers have taken great strides toward more environmentally and socially sensitive use of the trails. It is also the responsibility of hikers to make an extra effort to get along with other trail users. If hikers use common sense and follow the basic rules of courtesy, everyone will benefit and more fully enjoy the trail. If hikers don't reciprocate, they may turn into the dreaded inconsiderate backcountry blockhead (see sidebar). Don't let this happen to you!

Mountain bikers heading toward Watson Lake: Note the forest fire in the distance.

Sharing the Trail with Horses

While horseback riding can cause more damage to trails than any other use, equestrians account for a smaller percentage of trail users. Many equestrians, too, are actively involved in trail maintenance and construction. In my experience, horseback riders are courteous and willing to work with other users to share the trails.

Depending on individual circumstances and as a practical matter, all users should yield to each other. In general, hikers should yield to horses, while mountain bikers must yield to both hikers and horses: In other words, horses have the right-of-way on the trail. In the mid-1990s an article appeared in the Tahoe Rim Trail newsletter written by Sonja Willits, a woman with years of experience riding horses on Sierra trails. Willits did a good job of explaining trail use from the horse's point of view. With her permission, I've summarized the main points below.

- *A horse believes that everything will eat it until proven otherwise.* The first instinct of many horses is to run away, which can endanger both horse and rider, as well as anyone in the flight path who could get trampled or knocked off the trail. It is the job of all humans—equestrians, hikers, and mountain bikers—to assure the horse that no harm is intended.

- *When you are approaching a horse from behind, be sure to talk to the rider.* Talking calmly lets the horse know that you are not something that will hurt it. A bike that comes speeding up from behind a horse can severely frighten it. Be particularly cautious when rounding blind corners—horse riders often can't hear you coming.

- *When you see a horse coming toward you on the trail, talk to the rider.* Again, this soothes the horse and assures it that you are not a threat.

- *When approaching a horse going down a hill, pull over to the downhill slope of the trail and allow it to pass.* Spooked horses often want to go uphill.

- *If you are in a group of more than one biker or hiker, encourage everyone to move to the same side of the trail when you encounter horses.* Horses can feel trapped between you if you are standing on either side of the trail. An entrapped horse is not a good thing.

- *Wait to change clothes, repack your backpack, or make any sudden moves until the horses have passed.* While you are stopped, waiting for a horse to go by, it may seem perfectly fine to take off a shirt or rearrange things. As far as the horse is concerned, your movement and changed appearance may add to its feelings of being threatened.

Most horseback riders will move off the trail when it is easy for them to do so. They don't expect hikers and bike riders to give way all the time, particularly when the trail is especially narrow or precarious. However, it is the job of bike riders and hikers to step to the side first, and it is important to have a basic understanding of horse and rider psychology in order to be a conscientious sharer of the trail.

✓ Tim's Quick Tips for How to Be an Inconsiderate Backcountry Blockhead

✓ Make a lot of noise.

✓ While people are relaxing and enjoying the quiet at a mountain lake, yell at your friends on the other side.

✓ Let your dogs bark; when they take a swim, let them shake off on people you don't know.

✓ While you are walking along on the trail, talk loudly so that everyone within a half mile can hear you.

✓ If you are camping, make lots of noise late at night and again early in the morning. When you are in the quiet woods, it's party time!

✓ Loud stereos especially appeal to your average nature lover.

✓ Camp or sit close to other people. When you encounter a solitary person at a beautiful mountain lake, they obviously need some companionship and nonstop chatter.

✓ Don't worry about your garbage; someone else will pick it up. Anyway, it should biodegrade in a couple thousand years. Leave things in your campsite so that everyone knows you were there. It's a way to mark the good spots.

✓ Stay on the trail in people's way when they are trying to get by. If people are riding up a hill, stand in their way so that they have to get off their bikes; they will enjoy struggling to get back in their pedals on a steep hill.

✓ When you are walking or riding along the trail, ignore someone else who wants to pass. What's the hurry?

✓ Wash your dishes and clean your fish in streams and lakes. Fish thrive on detergent and consider bits of processed cheese great delicacies.

✓ Feed the animals. That way you help train them to get food from the next hiker who comes along. Backpackers get to practice the art of keeping animals out of their packs in the middle of the night. You can train some chipmunks and squirrels so well that they will practically jump into your lap to get a snack. While they can carry bubonic plague, the risk is a small price for well-trained squirrels.

✓ Leaving food out at night for bears is even more fun. The sound of a bear rampaging through your camp gives you a better rush than a double espresso.

Weather, Water, and When to Go

Some basic knowledge about the weather and water availability in the Lake Tahoe area and along its Rim Trail will help you plan a safe and enjoyable trip. All outdoor recreational activities in the Sierra are greatly affected by weather conditions. Of particular relevance is how much precipitation, usually in the form of snow, occurred the previous winter. Sierra Nevada winters come in a wide variety of sizes and time frames. In some years, it begins to snow in October and doesn't stop until June. After a year like that, hiking on dry land is out of the question until the middle of July in most areas. The following winter may not see snow until late January and then make up for it by dropping a lot of snow through May (a great year for late fall hiking). One season might have early heavy snow, followed by light snow, and then warm temperatures after February: This seasonal shift bodes well for those who want to get into the woods early to enjoy great wildflower displays and decent water availability.

Snowpack

The areas of highest elevation around Lake Tahoe often receive more than 600 inches of snow annually. Several factors determine whether the place you want to go will be out of the snow in the spring or summer, and some general rules govern the area's snowpack. Winter storms arrive primarily from the west, leaving lots of snow near the Sierra Crest. There is less snow as you travel farther east from the mountaintops. The west side of Lake Tahoe

Winter Wonderland

The winter landscape of the Sierra Nevada is both serene and pristine, with a beauty that you rarely find in the summer. In the winter, a soft white blanket covers the world with cold sparkles reflecting the blue sky. Walking or skiing through new fallen snow, you will find the rarest of gifts—peace and true quiet. In addition to the heavy snowfall in winter, you will also have some sunny winter days that provide wonderful opportunities to get out and enjoy all that deep white powder.

Although many people prefer to enjoy the mountains and woods in winter, it can be a more challenging and dangerous time. Unpredictable weather, unsigned trails, and other snow-related hazards are among the risk factors with which you should become familiar. Observe the weather and snow conditions. If the weather is getting bad, be smart, turn around and get out. Continually check your surroundings, observe familiar peaks, creeks, and other landmarks that will allow you to get back to your starting point if you are in a blizzard. Some of the most powerful blizzards can quickly become life-threatening. If you learn about mountain winter conditions and take a few simple precautions, much of the trail and areas in the Lake Tahoe area are great for winter snowshoeing or cross-country skiing.

Land Without Visible Trails

The fact that the Tahoe Rim Trail is not signed for winter creates challenges for even the most experienced traveler. Many popular winter spots may have tracks from the people who were there before you, but there are no real trails. You must follow landforms and head for saddles, mountaintops, or flats. Often, you may be heading in a general direction instead of to an exact spot. Know where you are and where you have been, and don't hesitate to follow your own tracks back out to where you began. It becomes even more important to have a map and follow it. Learn how to use a compass.

Dehydration

Drinking too little water is another serious risk when you are hiking, snowshoeing, snowboarding, or cross-country skiing. With all that snow around, you still need to remember to drink. When the weather is colder, people tend to drink less even though they may actually need as much water as they would on a hot day. While you are at it, eat. You'll need the energy.

Hypothermia and Frostbite

When the body's core temperature is seriously reduced as a result of exposure to cold and moisture, hypothermia can result. It is a serious condition, aggravated by cold wind and sudden climate changes. The symptoms of hypothermia include shivering, loss of coordination and the ability to do simple tasks, and disorientation and confusion. The treatment is based on common sense. First, get the victim out of the wind and elements. Prevent heat loss by getting the victim into warm, dry clothes (you should be carrying extra clothing in your pack). Get the victim into a sleeping bag, if you have one, and climb in to add your body heat (although, be careful as this approach may lower your own body temperature). Give the victim warm liquids and high carbohydrate foods.

Frostbite is the freezing of body tissues because of prolonged exposure to cold. The most susceptible areas to frostbite are the feet, hands, ears, and face. Prevention is key for both hypothermia and frostbite. Remember a few simple rules: Eat high-energy foods and drink plenty of liquids. Stay rested. Wear the right clothing and bring layers. Don't do something that will get you wet, and get out of the woods if you do get wet on a cold and windy day. Bring an extra set of clothes in case you get wet.

Avalanches

Understanding how avalanches occur and how to avoid them is too big a topic for this book, but a few words of warning can help you avoid a tragedy. Remember that you are most vulnerable to an avalanche when you are on moderately steep slopes (very steep slopes may not hold enough snow to avalanche), the lee side of mountains, or in gullies. Unstable snow conditions most often occur during or right after a storm; the bigger the storm, the bigger the risk. If you plan to do a lot of backcountry travel, take a Level One Avalanche Course, which will teach you how to determine avalanche risk, and how to work with beacons and probes to rescue those who have been caught in an avalanche. For more information or to obtain an updated avalanche danger report go to **www.avalanche.org** or **www. sierraavalanchecenter.org.**

Sunburn

The bright sun makes the snow even more beautiful and white. At the end of the day you have beautiful memories and one heck of a case of sunburn. Snow reflects the sun's rays like water and can burn your skin quickly. Use sunscreen and wear sunglasses to protect your eyes.

> ❄ **Tim's Quick Tips: Avoiding Winter Weather Risks**
>
> ❋ Keep an eye on the weather forecasts until right before you leave. Many great weather sources exist, including local radio and television stations (KCRA-Sacramento, and KOLO-Reno are two of them); The Weather Channel (on cable television); and, these websites—**www. wunderground.com** and **www. writeonrex.com**—are also useful.
>
> ❋ Before setting out, let someone know where you are going and when you plan to return.
>
> ❋ Bring extra layers of clothing. The weather may change for the worse even if the forecast calls for nice weather.
>
> ❋ Do not venture out unless you know how to navigate without a visible trail.
>
> ❋ Use a compass and map.
>
> ❋ Bring your survival kit!
>
> ❋ Drink lots of water.
>
> ❋ Avoid situations that cause hypothermia and frostbite.

Guided Winter Hikes

The Tahoe Rim Trail Association runs a program of guided snowshoe hikes during the winter months. Past trips have included full moon jaunts in Tahoe Meadows and daytime hikes into Page Meadows. For more information go to **www.tahoerimtrail.org.**

Packing and Dressing for Winter Weather

Aside from sunblock, be sure to carry a basic survival kit. Your kit should include the following items:

- Two large plastic garbage bags (to be used as a poncho or emergency shelter in bad weather)
- Waterproof matches
- Candle
- Metal cup for melting snow
- Duct tape for repairs (can be wrapped around a ski pole)
- Cocoa or other powdered mix
- Cell phone (but don't count on using it)

You have three goals when it comes to clothing yourself for outdoor winter adventures: keep dry, keep warm, and keep cool. To accomplish these goals, wear or pack clothing made of synthetic fibers. They are lightweight and whisk moisture away from your body, which will help to keep you warm. Bring several lightweight layers of clothes, including a waterproof outer shell; it will help you stay dry but allow you to remain cool if the temperature turns warm. Wear a sturdy pair of waterproof boots with two pairs of socks: a thin inner layer of socks made of synthetic fiber and a thicker outer layer of wool or synthetic fiber. Wear water-resistant pants, such as those designed for cross-country skiing; over them, wear a waterproof shell if you are snowshoeing or traveling through deep snow. A hat is essential, whether it is a baseball cap on a warm day or a warm fleece hat on a cold day.

And don't forget gloves; the style depends on the conditions and activity you are doing. If it is warm and you will be strenuously cross-country skiing, lightweight ski gloves are fine. If you are out hiking or snowshoeing on a cold snowy day, bring a thicker, warmer pair of gloves.

The Great Ski Race

When (and Where) to Go

Winter to Spring

For those who love the snow and winter sports, there are a number of places that are especially attractive and challenging for winter activities. Here are a few of the best spots:

Page Meadows

The easiest way to access Page Meadows in winter is through the Talmont Estates subdivision. From Tahoe City, go 2 miles south on Highway 89 to Pine Avenue. Turn right, and then right again on Tahoe Park Heights. Go to the top of the hill, and take Big Pine, the middle of three roads. Follow Big Pine to Silvertip and turn left. There is limited parking available at the end of Silvertip. From the end of the road, head west a few hundred yards to the first of several meadows. The area around Page Meadows is especially popular for cross-country skiing and snowshoeing. The terrain is mostly level, perfect for beginners. The meadows are beautiful on a sunny day or at night when the moon is full.

Tahoe Meadows

Located on the south side of Highway 431, the meadow is great for a beginner on either skis or snowshoes. From Incline Village, drive 7 miles up Highway 431, the Mt. Rose Highway. Here, you will see a large treeless area on your right. Park along the road. Both the large open meadow and its surrounding forest are popular for winter sports; in fact, on a weekend you might find this area too crowded. Head south up through the trees to a saddle for extraordinary lake views. You could well be dazzled by lodgepole and whitebark pines covered with hoarfrost.

On the north side of the highway at Tahoe Meadows, the TRT climbs toward the radio tower and Mt. Rose, another excellent area to ski or snowshoe. While this route can get quite steep and difficult near the top, the views of Mt. Rose and Lake Tahoe from the radio tower are inspiring.

Tahoe Cross-Country Ski Area

Located on Dollar Hill about 2 miles east of Tahoe City along Highway 28, Tahoe Cross-Country is the venue for the Great Ski Race from Tahoe City to Truckee, which crosses the TRT. This wonderful area provides 65 kilometers of trails through the forests between Mount Watson and Tahoe City. Many of this Nordic center's trails are popular with mountain bikers and hikers in the summer. Contact Tahoe Cross-Country at (530) 583-5475 or visit **www.tahoexc.org.**

Kirkwood Cross-Country Ski Area

Kirkwood is located 30 miles south of South Lake Tahoe on Highway 88. It has a network of more than 50 miles of trails with spectacular views of the Carson Pass and Kirkwood area. For more information, call (209) 258-7248 or visit **www.kirkwood.com/ site/cross-country/xc-center.**

For additional information on winter trail use, pick up a copy of *Snowshoe Trails of Tahoe* by Mike White, also published by Wilderness Press. The Tahoe Nordic Search and Rescue Team has all kinds of valuable information, and they are the guys and gals you will be really happy to see if you get lost in the snow. Some of the information in this section comes from the Tahoe Nordic Search and Rescue team's winter awareness brochure, *A Guide to Winter Preparedness and Survival.* To obtain a copy or for more information, call (530) 581-4038. Above all else, if you have a phone, in an emergency call 911.

Summer to Fall

Summer and early fall at Tahoe are mostly sunny, warm, and glorious. Nevertheless, afternoon thunderstorms do come up. Some summers may have no thunderstorms, while in other years, they may occur almost daily. Usually storms are scattered, developing— sometimes out of a clear blue sky—during mid- to late afternoon when the temperatures are warm and a great deal of tropical moisture has moved in from the south. Keep your eye on any large, high, darkening clouds moving rather quickly in your general direction. Better yet, check out the weather information channel or local weather broadcasts and plan accordingly. You can also visit **www.wunderground.com** or **www.writeonrex.com.**

The chance of a thunderstorm need not thwart or curtail your plans, but do bring your rain gear. Sometimes a storm moves swiftly through a specific area and drops only a little rain before it passes. However, if it gets exciting and lightning starts to flash, get out as quickly as possible, especially if you are on an exposed peak, near bodies of water, or under tall trees. Avoid areas of high exposure, such as the top of a pass. I can tell you from personal experience that Dicks Pass, for example, is not a good place to be in a thunderstorm. Avoid the urge to take shelter under a solitary tree in open lands. If you cannot get out of the woods in time, stay in the forest in an area of similar-sized trees. While lightning can be scary and dangerous, it is also important to remember that people are rarely struck by a lightning bolt. Absent a bit of very bad luck, if you take reasonable precautions you should be fine.

Water

Much of the Tahoe Rim Trail is located along ridgetops, a perfect situation for enjoying the sublime views of Lake Tahoe and the surrounding mountains. However, its rim location results in a shortage of water along many sections of the trail, especially on the sections along the east shore. Plan ahead and make sure you have enough water to get you through the section you will be hiking. On hot summer days, you will need at least 2 to 3 quarts of water. Water is an especially important issue to consider if you plan to thru-hike the entire TRT.

Be sure to avoid drinking any untreated water in the Sierra Nevada. Giardia, a microorganism that occurs in many bodies of water here, can cause havoc in your intestines. To prevent giardia or other bugs from getting into your system, be sure to filter, boil, or chemically treat any water that you draw from a natural source.

In each section of the trail described in chapter 6 (page 69), additional specific water information is provided.

Fun for All
and All for Fun:
A User's Guide
to the Tahoe Rim Trail

During spring, summer, and fall, many types of users enjoy the Tahoe Rim Trail; each has particular needs, but all have the same general goal of having fun, enjoying nature, and challenging themselves on the trail. Because one user's mode of transport on the trail—whether it is a pair of legs, a pair of wheels, or four strong horse hooves—can affect another's, this chapter focuses on the different types of users and offer tips and suggestions for a mutually safe and pleasant journey.

A Hiking Paradise

Most people who buy this book probably enjoy hiking already and know the basics: Carry plenty of water; wear comfortable boots or shoes; take a map, guidebook, and sunscreen; and bring extra clothes in case of a change in the weather. Chapter 6 (page 69) has complete descriptions of each section of the TRT, plus information about short spur trails that hikers can add to customize their outings. Every section of the trail offers something unique, whether it is the scenery or the specific challenge of the route.

To get the most out of your journey, take care of a few simple things before you leave. Most importantly, tell someone where you are going and when you expect to be back, and then check in when you return. Although the TRT is not as isolated as a lot of backcountry areas, you may still be alone on many parts of it. It is only common sense to leave information with a friend or family member about your general whereabouts. Much of the Tahoe Rim Trail is used primarily by daytime users, so late in the day you are most likely to be alone on the trail. The checklist of key things to remember in the sidebar on page 49 will help you plan your Tahoe Rim Trail trek.

Backpacking and Camping

Why not hike the whole Tahoe Rim Trail? Depending on how strong a hiker you are, it takes anywhere from ten days to three weeks to encircle Lake Tahoe on this route. (Such a hike is called a "thru-hike.") Two weeks would be a comfortable period (although two weeks of backpacking and comfort are not usually used in the same sentence). Since the TRT is a loop trail, you could start anywhere and end up right back where you began.

A backpacking trip of this length requires some logistical planning. Your primary concerns will be where to camp and where to get water and additional food. Camping is allowed without restrictions everywhere on the Tahoe Rim Trail except in Desolation Wilderness where you must obtain a permit. For more information, call (530) 573-2674. Although permits are not required in Lake Tahoe Nevada State Park, camping there is limited to two primitive campgrounds, each with a pit toilet and picnic tables. The Marlette Campground also provides water through a hand-operated well. For more information, call (775) 831-0494.

To find out where else you can camp, refer to the trail descriptions in Chapter 6 (page 69). For water availability, review the Heads Up section at the beginning of each trail description. If you are hiking in late summer or fall, keep in mind that some of the water may have dried up. If you come to a major water source in the fall, fill up, but be sure to boil, filter, or treat the water before drinking it.

The good news (or bad depending on your perspective) is that a lot of people live at Lake Tahoe who have built communities with stores that carry every amenity you could possibly need.

Road Crossings and Drop-Off Points

You can design your backpacking trip so that you can pick up food and supplies at various locations and trailheads along the way. Between the stops where you may have arranged to meet friends, you will need water. Here is a summary of the road crossings and communities along the TRT.

❀ Tim's Top Tips for Backcountry Hikers

❀ Bring more water than you think you will need.

❀ Don't drink the water in lakes and streams unless you boil, filter, or treat it.

❀ Carry a first-aid kit. If you take something out, don't forget to restock it.

❀ Dress in layers. Don't wear cotton except on hot dry days in midsummer.

❀ Wear good hiking boots or comfortable athletic shoes. Some hikers prefer the newer high-quality hiking sandals.

❀ Wear hiking socks made of synthetic material or wool *not* cotton.

❀ Bring enough clothes; temperatures can change quickly.

❀ Bring rain gear—the weather can change rapidly in the Sierra.

❀ Carry and use sunscreen.

❀ Start out early when it is still cool and there are fewer people on the trail.

❀ Bring a map and this guidebook. A good field guide is also useful.

❀ Tell someone where you're going and when you expect to return; check in when you return.

❀ If your knees hurt when you hike, try using trekking poles. They can make a significant difference when you hike downhill and help to balance you when you need to scramble over a rocky section of trail.

❀ If you have recently come from a much lower altitude, take time to acclimate to a higher altitude before you set off.

Tahoe City (Sections 1 and 8)

The trail route goes right through Tahoe City, a good midway stopping point if you started your trip at Echo Summit or Kingsbury Grade. As you cross the road from one section of the trail to the next, you will be within 100 yards of a supermarket and within half a mile of several motels. The latter are often booked in the summer; call ahead and warn them to have the showers ready. Tahoe City is loaded with outfitters who will be happy to sell you any equipment you may have forgotten or need to replace. Check out Alpenglow located near the trail on North Lake Blvd., the main road that goes through the center of town.

Kings Beach (Sections 1 and 2)

The trail crosses Highway 267 at 2.75 miles northwest of Kings Beach. A supermarket, with most of the supplies you may need, is located near the intersection of Highway 267 and Highway 28. Outfitter Tahoe Mountain Sports can be found in the middle of Kings Beach. This road crossing is a good place for a friend to drop off food or water, or you could leave a stash of water here in advance. Very little water is available on the section of trail between Tahoe City and Brockway Summit; when you cross Highway 267, the next water source is a spring beyond Mud Lake or Gray Lake, both more than 10 miles away. *The spring may run dry by fall, so don't count on it.*

Incline Village (Sections 2 and 3)

The TRT crosses Highway 431 at 8 miles above Incline Village, another place to meet your wonderful friends who have brought you fresh supplies. Be sure to load up on water at Ophir Creek, about a mile along the trail after you cross Highway 431. The next water source is at the Marlette Campground, 14 miles to the south.

Spooner Summit to Highway 50 (Sections 3 and 4)

There are no towns nearby, but this first road crossing in 23 miles may be a good place to stop and get replenished by those now great friends of yours (your "trail angels").

Daggett Pass (Sections 4 and 5)

There are no amenities where the road crosses SR 207 (Kingsbury Grade), but you can access the Tramway Market by crossing North Benjamin Road to the North Dagget Loop and then walking up the Dagget Summit Connector to Tramway Road. After visiting the market you can continue up the Tramway Market paved road to the Stagecoach Kingsbury Grade South Trailhead. At 2.6 miles south of Kingsbury Grade, you meet a junction where the Van Sickle Trail takes you past beautiful lake views in 3.3 miles to South Lake Tahoe, just above the casinos. Here you will find Heavenly Village with a supermarket and a host of other amenities, including lodging.

Highway 89, Big Meadow Trailhead (Sections 5 and 6)

You have just hiked 23 grueling miles when you get to the road where there is nothing except a bathroom. Use it. This crossing is another good drop-off point where your loyal friends can bring you food acquired in nearby South Lake Tahoe or Meyers. If your friends don't show up or you have an emergency, Meyers is about 5.3 miles downhill from the trailhead.

Echo Summit and Resort (Sections 6 and 7)

After 17.5 more miles past Big Meadow Trailhead, you reach the Echo Lakes Chalet, (530) 659-7207, which has a store. Stock up because Barker Pass Road is 33 miles north. The chalet has a seasonal post office open during the summer months where you can pick up a package of food that you were smart enough to mail to yourself before you left on your excursion. Or you can mail food to the next town post office, Tahoe City, 49 miles away. Echo Lakes Chalet sells excellent sandwiches and ice cream, both highlights when I arrived there on day eleven of a TRT thru-hike.

Barker Pass (Sections 7 and 8)

This remote road crossing is more than 11 miles from Tahoe City via Barker Pass Road and Highway 89, but it could work as a drop-off point in a pinch. The road is closed in the winter and remains closed until the snow has melted.

Ward Creek Road (Section 8)

The trail crosses this road halfway between Barker Pass and Tahoe City. If necessary, you could ask someone to meet you at this road crossing to supply moral support and give you the news of the day, but Tahoe City is only 5 more miles away.

While depending upon your friends to assist with your thru-hiking plans is certainly desirable, if that doesn't work out you may have to make arrangements yourself. Fending for yourself means caching water ahead of time—placing a gallon or two near the trailhead a few days before your departure—in a few of the driest sections. It also means either mailing food packages to yourself or picking up food along the way. Tahoe City or South Lake Tahoe, with great outdoor stores and several supermarkets a short distance off the trail, are your best bets for resupplying on the trail.

What to Bring in Your Backpack

My good friend and hiking buddy Shannon Raborn hiked the entire 2,100 miles of the Appalachian Trail that runs between Georgia and Maine. When she told me what to bring on a spring, summer, or fall backpacking trip in the Sierra, I listened. I thank Shannon for her helpful contributions to the following list, which we wrote together.

First, you will want to organize your pack by the object's use. Remember, the less weight and space taken up, the better off you will be as you carry it down (and up and down again) the trail.

Clothes

Pack hiking shorts, shirts (made of lightweight, preferably synthetic fibers), warm fleece shirt, rain shell, several pairs of socks, Tevas, Crocs, or water socks (for around camp), baseball hat, warm pants or convertible pants that are shorts during the day and pants at night. If it will be very cold or you are cold-natured, bring a fleece hat and gloves.

Toiletries

Bring a toothbrush, toothpaste, vitamins and medications, sunscreen, toilet paper, biodegradable all-purpose soap, and a scrubby sponge for cleaning pots, pans, and your hands. Pack any scented products in a scent-proof container, and remember to store them in a bear canister when you sleep at night.

Camping Supplies

Bring a first-aid kit, tent, rope, Thermarest pad, sleeping bag (lightweight is best), backpacking pillow (a luxury, but it feels SOOOO good!), camp stove (I like Jet Boil's all-in-one pot and stove with gas canisters), gas for your stove, water filter and/or iodine tablets, water bottles, Camelbak or other water storage container (which allows you to carry large amounts of water, necessary on the dryer sections of the TRT), trowel (pooper scooper), lighter and/or matches, pot and pan kit, bowl, cup, utensils (spoon or fork), small sharp knife, compass, headlamp or flashlight, map, heavyweight garbage bags (to keep things dry in case of rain), duct tape, field guides, this book of course, and a camera.

If you are "camping light," the weather forecast does not call for rain, and it is past mosquito season (late summer), you could forego the tent and rain fly. If you do not mind going without cooked food, you can also eliminate the stove, fuel, and pots and pans. Keeping your clothes to a minimum is another technique to lower weight, but be sure to not cut out something you may need to stay warm and dry.

Bear Canisters

In areas with lots of bears (anywhere near Lake Tahoe), bear canisters are essential. Canisters not only work well at keeping out small animals such as squirrels and marmots, but they can serve as a chair or as a washtub for doing your laundry.

Food

Plan what you need, but keep it light. Remember that John Muir took only a pocket full of biscuits with him! Freeze-dried dinners are tasty, but they can be expensive for a long trip. I especially like the ones that require only hot water. Some recommended food items are: instant oatmeal, pasta, couscous, soup, energy bars, gorp or trail mix, bagels, salami, hard cheese, avocadoes, tortillas with stuffing such as cheese or cooked chicken, crackers, hot chocolate or coffee, fruit packages, cereal, powdered milk, cookies, and tea.

Yippee! Mountain Biking

When the Tahoe Rim Trail was first built, mountain biking was prohibited on it. As time went by and regulations eased, about half the trail has become open to mountain bikers. It is important to understand that the Tahoe Rim Trail is really only suitable for intermediate and advanced riders. Most sections are quite difficult and technical, so riders should make sure they are capable of riding the section before setting out.

The areas closed to bikers include the approximate 50 miles of the route that overlap with the Pacific Crest Trail. Bikes are also forbidden in the wilderness areas: Desolation Wilderness and Mt. Rose Wilderness. Also, bikes are prohibited on a section of trail going north from Spooner Summit past Snow Valley Peak to Hobart Road and the trail to Galena Falls from the Mt. Rose Trailhead. Bikes are permitted on the rest of the TRT.

For detailed descriptions of each section of the trail, directions to trailheads, and special sidebars applying to bikers, refer to individual trail descriptions. Here's a summary of which sections you can or cannot ride on (these are also shown on the maps).

Section 1: Tahoe City to Brockway   Riding is allowed on the entire section.

🚴 Tim's Top Tips for Mountain Bikers

🚴 Ride only where bicycles are permitted.

🚴 Wear your helmet.

🚴 Speed is your friend. Hitting the brakes too hard or going too slowly over a rocky section can send you flying over the bars. With a little speed you can bounce right over the rocks. Of course, if you fall, the rule has now changed to "Speed is your friend, until it isn't."

🚴 To prevent undue erosion, avoid wet, muddy areas.

🚴 Spring and fall temperatures, which are bearable when you're hiking, get bone-chilling as you cruise downhill at 20 miles an hour. When it's cold, wear a warm ski hat under your helmet, warm socks, and lots of layers. Your legs will be pumping so they won't get as cold, but the wind goes right to your neck and through those bike shoes.

🚴 Wear bike shoes, bike shorts, and bike shirts; they are well designed to make your ride more enjoyable.

🚴 Wear a Camelbak or other water-hydration system. Mountain biking is strenuous exercise, and a water bottle isn't sufficient on a warm day. Additionally, a Camelbak lets you drink without stopping and keeps the water colder throughout the whole ride.

🚴 When riding downhill, lift your bottom slightly off the seat, lean back gently, don't grip the handlebars too tightly, and flow down that awesome single track. (Don't forget to yippee!)

🚴 Learn how to fix a flat and do minor repairs on your bike; bring a spare inner tube.

🚴 Scrapes and cuts are common while biking; carry a small, light first-aid kit in your pack. One good brand is the Optimist by Adventure Medical Kits.

Section 2: Brockway to Mt. Rose Mountain biking is allowed between Brockway Summit and the Mt. Rose Wilderness boundary, a distance of about 7 miles. If you start from the Tahoe Meadows end, there are two trails, one that allows mountain bikes and one that does not. Follow the instructions for that section. Either way you can go only 4 miles to the Relay Peak Tower on your bike.

Section 3: Tahoe Meadows to Spooner Summit Mountain biking is allowed between Tahoe Meadows and Hobart Road, which is 14.3 miles (for the section between Tahoe Meadows and

Tunnel Creek Road, which is 9.2 miles, mountain biking is allowed only on even days of the month). At Hobart Road, a detour is available down to Marlette Lake and then out to Spooner Lake via North Canyon Road.

Section 4: Spooner Summit to Kingsbury Grade This entire section is open to bikes.

Section 5: Kingsbury Grade to Big Meadow This entire section is open to bikes, but much of it is very difficult.

Section 6: Big Meadow to the Pacific Crest Trail Bikes are allowed from the Big Meadow Trailhead for about 5 miles to where the Tahoe Rim Trail meets the Pacific Crest Trail in Meiss Meadows. Bikes are prohibited on the PCT.

Section 7: Echo Summit to Barker Pass Bikes are not allowed on this entire section, which overlaps with the PCT.

Section 8: Barker Pass to Tahoe City The first 5 miles are on the PCT; bikes are prohibited on the PCT. From Twin Peaks to Tahoe City, bikes are allowed.

Getting Horsey on the TRT

For most horseback riders, the entire Tahoe Rim Trail is a great place to ride. While some equestrians may find a few sections difficult (Desolation Wilderness and an area south of Barker Pass especially), almost all of it is very good for riding. Water is a concern on much of the trail, especially on the east shore. If you plan to ride on the TRT, be sure to read through trail descriptions for detailed information. While on the trail, watch out for other users. Horses are supposed to be given the right-of-way, but be alert and cautious just the same. Horses are fairly rare on the TRT—other users may not expect to see them. Many experts suggest equestrians always wear helmets. Learn the trail ahead of time, and be sure to maintain a comfortable pace for yourself and your horse. Stay on the trail to protect the fragile environment. Two other issues

Horses at Dardanelles Lake

that equestrians must consider before embarking on a ride along the TRT: where to park and where to camp.

Where to Park the Trailer

Tahoe City

There are two parking locations close to the trailheads. Both can be crowded with narrow access. The first is at the 64 Acres (Truckee River Access) parking lot located on Highway 89, 0.25 mile south of its intersection with Highway 28 in Tahoe City. From here, you can ride along a paved road for a short distance and then meet the TRT heading toward Page Meadows.

The second Tahoe City parking spot is located at the Fairway Community Center on Fairway Drive, directly across the street from the Tahoe Rim Trail section that goes from Tahoe City to Watson Lake and then on to Brockway Summit. From the Tahoe City "Y" (the intersection of Highways 89 and 28) go 0.2 mile on Highway 89 toward Truckee and turn right on Fairway Drive. Drive 0.2 mile to the Fairway Community Center on the right.

If you park at 64 Acres and ride toward Watson Lake, it can be challenging because you must cross a busy bike bridge, walk on a congested section of bike trail, and then cross Highway 89 to walk 0.2 mile on Fairway Drive.

Brockway Summit

There are two parking areas available here. You can park along the road at the TRT parking area, 0.5 mile east of Brockway Summit, which has room for only a few cars and requires you to unload your horse near a busy road. The second location is 0.2 mile past the top of Brockway Summit toward Truckee. On the right is a road leading up to Martis Peak. This is a great spot for horses, and from here you can ride your horse up the lightly traveled Martis Peak Road several miles until you meet the TRT.

Mt. Rose and Tahoe Meadows

The Tahoe Meadows Trailhead parking lot was designed for horses, but it may be congested on a busy day. If it is full, the meadow side of the road has a wide shoulder. After you park, follow the sign toward Brockway Summit or Spooner Summit. If you are heading toward Brockway Summit from this trailhead, use extreme caution since you will have to ride parallel to and then cross the very busy road to the trailhead. There is also limited parking at the Mt. Rose Trailhead.

Spooner Summit

Both trailheads on Spooner Summit have convenient places to park your trailer. It is best to park on the side of the road where you will begin your ride so that you do not have to cross Highway 50, a major highway with cars roaring by at high speed.

Kingsbury Grade, North

The north trailhead of Kingsbury Grade has room to park your trailer along this quiet subdivision road.

Kingsbury Grade, South

The large Heavenly Ski Area Stagecoach parking lot should provide plenty of room to park your horse trailer.

Big Meadow

The Big Meadow Parking lot has parking spots designed for horse trailers, but the access is quite narrow. Often the horse-trailer parking spots have been taken by cars in this crowded parking area (if you do not have a horse, give those with horses a break and park in the other spaces if they are available). The parking lot has some challenging, winding, sharp turns. If you are heading toward Freel Peak, you can park along the road near the Grass Lake Trailhead and then use this connector trail.

Echo Summit

At the top of the summit on the south side of the road there is a large snow park that makes for a great spot to park your trailer. From here, you can ride across the parking lot and head south or follow the trail north to Lower Echo Lake. There is also parking at Lower Echo Lake, although it can be full to overflowing on summer weekends.

Barker Pass

There is plenty of parking space available at the top of Barker Pass. From here, you can head in either direction on the Tahoe Rim Trail. The paved road up to Barker Pass is a good one but has a few narrow, twisting turns.

Places to Horse Camp

When looking for a place to camp when you are backpacking, your primary considerations are finding water and a pretty spot. When you have a horse, another concern enters the picture: Where do you find grass for your horses without destroying a beautiful meadow? Equestrians should bring their own horse feed instead of relying on unpredictable and fragile grass and meadowlands.

Some of the good camping spots for horses include:

- **Watson Lake**

- **Ophir Creek:** Go straight at the TRT and Ophir Creek Trail junction to a nice spot near the creek but out of Tahoe Meadows. You are now on Ophir Creek Trail but still close to the TRT.

- **Star Lake**

- **Armstrong Pass:** Take the Armstrong Pass connector trail down to the dirt road and a nearby stream. The dry meadow area is known as Horse Meadow.

- **Meiss Meadows and the area near Showers Lake**

- **Desolation Wilderness:** See permit information in Chapter 1 (page 6).

- **Ward Canyon, below Twin Peaks**

- **Robie Equestrian Park:** This special 160-acre wilderness equestrian park serves as the staging area for the annual Tevis Cup 100-mile horse ride from Tahoe to Auburn. While not on the Tahoe Rim Trail, the equestrian park is 3 miles from Watson Lake and has two trails with direct access to the TRT. Accessible by vehicle, it is a convenient place for horse camping or setting out for day rides. Livestock water, outhouse facilities, and ample parking are available. The park is open to day use throughout the summer. Reservations for overnight camping are needed in advance. Contact the Wendell and Inez Robie Foundation at P.O. Box 714, Foresthill, CA 95631, (530) 367-4332, **www.robiefoundation.org/park.htm.**

Goin' Fishin'

Rainbow trout, brook trout, brown trout, and cutthroat trout are the most common fish in the mountain lakes and streams around Lake Tahoe. In a few lakes, including Lake Tahoe itself, you will also find kokanee salmon and mackinaw trout (which has edged out the cutthroat in the lake). Most mountain lakes are stocked with fish on a regular basis, although there has been talk of ending the stocking program, especially in wilderness areas, which could greatly affect the mountain fishing experience.

Fishing on the Rim Trail is just like anywhere else: Anyone older than 16 must have a fishing license. To obtain a license, contact your local sporting goods store. If you have questions about fishing regulations in California, call the California Department of Fish and Game at (916) 358-2900. In Nevada, call the Nevada Division of Wildlife at (775) 688-1500.

Much of the Tahoe Rim Trail lies along the ridgelines surrounding the Lake Tahoe Basin. It is generally above the lake areas and the major streams that support fish populations. However, several locations along the trail are good for fishing, and a number of spur trails take you to good fishing sites. In general, since most of the lakes and streams are above the west shore, that is where the best fishing opportunities are. Since half the fun of fishing is discovering your own secret hole, I reveal only the more popular places below.

The best way to make sure that Tahoe area waterways continue to have fish is to practice the catch-and-release fishing technique. Create barbless hooks by smashing the barb on your hook with a pair of pliers. Once you catch the fish, treat them gently. Remove the hook while the fish is still in the water, and release it back into the environment where it belongs. If you are camping and really would enjoy a fish dinner, go ahead, but be sure to only take the fish you will eat (and don't clean the fish in the nearest lake or stream).

For more details about fishing in the Sierra, refer to *Sierra Trout Guide* by Ralph Cutter, published by Amato Publications. It provides a list of every lake in the Sierra and what kind of fish may be found there. Or check out Ralph's website at **www.fly line.com**. Another informative source is the *Desolation Wilderness Fishing Guide* by Jerome Yesavage, also published by Amato.

Desolation Wilderness and Western Rim

The area between Echo Lakes and Barker Pass has an abundance of fishable lakes. Explore the area, and you will find the best spots to fish.

Truckee River

In Tahoe City the TRT meets the Truckee River, a popular fishing spot. During summer months this area is also popular with rafters. It is best to fish in early morning or late afternoon, or you may catch a big raft instead of a trout.

North Shore

Watson Lake, which is a fairly shallow lake, is pretty much your only choice in this area. Two other lakes in the area, Gray Lake and Mud Lake, do not have fish and are sometimes not even lakes.

East Shore

Only a few lakes of any size exist on the east shore. Close to the trail and right off the highway is Spooner Lake, a catch-and-release fishing area only. Marlette Lake is also catch and release. Because the shallow Twin Lakes often dry up in late season, they lack fish, but Star Lake, at the base of Jobs Sister, has trout.

South Shore and Meiss Meadows Areas

In this area, the Upper Truckee River, Meiss Lake, Dardanelles Lake, Round Lake, and Showers Lake provide opportunities for fishing. In recent years Tahoe's native fish, the Lahontan cutthroat, has been reintroduced to these waters, and a zero limit, catch-and-release policy has been instituted.

Kids Like to Hike . . . Some Kids. . . Sometimes . . . and Not Too Far

The Tahoe Rim Trail is a challenging trail for grown-ups because it traverses terrain that has lots of elevation gain. Much of the trail is simply not suitable for younger children. There are, however, a few great destinations for family outings. Here are a few suggestions on my favorite places to take children. The complete route descriptions are in Chapter 6, page 69.

Mt. Rose and Tahoe Meadows Area

Near the top of the Mt. Rose Highway at Tahoe Meadows, the Tahoe Rim Trail has two trailheads and an interpretive trail. All three provide an opportunity for kids to learn about and enjoy the mountains. Each of these trailheads is located above 8000 feet, about 7.5 miles up Highway 431 from the intersection of Highway 28 and Highway 431 in Incline Village. They are all in the same vicinity or across the street from each other.

Tahoe Meadows Interpretative Trail

If you are coming from Incline Village on Highway 431, you will see a parking area and a building set down below the road on the right-hand side after about 7.5 miles. This area has a very easy, wheelchair- and stroller-accessible, 1.3-mile loop. The trail starts on the eastern edge of the lower parking area and winds through the meadow. It is a great spot for early summer wildflowers and a place where the little ones can stretch their legs. This is the easiest segment of the Tahoe Rim Trail and is suitable for very young children.

Take them before they grow up!

Tahoe Meadows to Spooner Summit

This hike starts from the western edge of the same parking lot as described just above. First, the trail traverses Tahoe Meadows and passes a display of wildflowers, a few small streams, and larger Ophir Creek—a playground for kids. Once you have crossed the meadow, the trail levels out and heads uphill, not too steeply, to the top of a saddle 1.7 miles from the trailhead. From the saddle, the trail levels off again and remains mostly level for several miles with only a few gentle up-and-down passages. The views of the lake are incredible, and numerous flat rock "armchairs" invite you to enjoy your lunch or a snack. Walk as far as you want, and then turn around. This area is also a great spot for someone who is learning how to cross-country snowshoe or ski.

Tahoe Meadows and Mt. Rose to Brockway Summit

From Incline Village on Highway 431, drive past the main Tahoe Meadows Trailhead on your right and go another 0.7 mile, where you reach the Mt. Rose and TRT Trailhead with restrooms and parking. For your family outing, hike up the trail. Lake Tahoe, Tahoe Meadows, and the mountains around the lake quickly come into view. In 2.5 miles of fairly easy walking you reach lovely Galena Falls where you reach a junction. A left turn takes you up to the top of the falls, where you can turn left and head to Snow Pond, or go straight ahead on new single track toward Relay Peak. From Snow Pond you can turn around, or follow the dirt road and mountain biking–friendly TRT section back to the trailhead for a 6-mile loop.

If you take the right turn toward the Mt. Rose Summit, at the bottom of the falls you will quickly cross two streams and find great mid-season wildflower displays.

Big Meadow Area

Drive 5.3 miles south of Meyers on Highway 89 to the Tahoe Rim Trail Big Meadow Trailhead. This trail heads northeast toward Kingsbury Grade, or south 5 miles to where the Tahoe Rim Trail intersects the Pacific Crest Trail. If your children are hearty, they may enjoy the hike south where, after about 3 miles and approximately 800 feet of elevation gain, you will reach Round Lake. Along the way, you traverse lovely Big Meadow. You will also encounter some huge volcanic rock formations. The lake itself is a great respite for the kids. (You could also take the spur trail to Dardanelles Lake, a beautiful lake 3.4 miles from the trailhead).

Echo Lakes Area

At Lower Echo Lake (see directions in Chapter 6, Section 7, page 157), you will find a store, a small marina, and a large parking facility. From the lake, your trail is the Tahoe Rim Trail, Tahoe-Yosemite Trail, and the Pacific Crest Trail all combined; it heads north. The first 2.5 miles are along the Lower and Upper Echo Lakes and provide great views of them. This trail has some fun up-and-down passages and rocky scrambles, perfect for any 10 year old.

At the end of 2.5 miles, you can continue on the trail, turn around, or take the Echo Lakes Water Taxi back to the Echo Lakes parking lot. The taxi is a small boat that travels back and forth across the lakes. It only operates seasonally, so be sure to check ahead for taxi times and to make sure it is running. The taxi pier is a great place for a swim while you are waiting for the boat. Late in the summer the lake level drops too low to allow passage for the taxi between Lower and Upper Echo Lakes. For more information about the Echo Lakes Water Taxi, contact Echo Lakes Chalet at (530) 659-7207.

Another option is to take the taxi to the end of the two lakes and cut out 2.5 miles of a trip to Lake of the Woods or Lake Aloha. If you take the water taxi, it is only about 3 miles to Lake of the Woods and 3.5 miles to the eastern edge of Lake Aloha. I found Lake Aloha to be a perfect spot to take my child on a backpacking trip. Be prepared for a hearty climb of about 1000 feet through rocky terrain.

Page Meadows Area

The Page Meadows area can be approached from several different directions and is an excellent and easy place to take the kids on a hike. The easiest way into the area is through the back of the Talmont Estates and Twin Peaks subdivision. Take Highway 89 south about 2 miles from Tahoe City. Turn right on Pine Avenue. In about 0.2 mile, turn right on Tahoe Park Heights. Follow Tahoe Park Heights to the top of the hill and then take Big Pine, the middle of three roads. Continue on Big Pine for about 0.25 mile to Silvertip Drive where you turn left. Follow Silvertip to the end of the road, and park where you see a sign that reads SKI PARKING. A dirt road heads west from the end of the road. Follow it down the hill straight ahead until you pass a sharp left-hand turn. Just after the turn, a single-track trail heads off to the right and arrives at the first meadow in about 100 yards. Follow the edge of the meadow until you see a trail heading left (west) through the meadow. From here you can start exploring. The trail goes by several big meadows. The meadows provide tremendous mountain views, great wildflowers in the summer, and lots of aspen trees making it prime for fall colors. Bring a picnic lunch and a Frisbee and have at it with the kids. Avoid trampling the fragile meadow at least until late summer or fall when it has had a chance to dry out.

Ward Canyon Area

On Highway 89, drive 2.4 miles south of Tahoe City, past Sunnyside Resort to Pineland Drive on the right. In 0.4 mile it becomes Twin Peaks Drive. Stay on the left at the Y, and in about 0.1 mile the road becomes Ward Creek Boulevard. Take this about 1.5 miles to a TAHOE RIM TRAIL sign on your left where the trail begins. Follow the old road as it parallels the largely unseen Ward Creek for the next 3 miles. Go as far as you want and then turn around. The trail eventually leads rather steeply up to Twin Peaks, but that would be a long haul for the little ones. The first 3 miles, however, are a gentle uphill with lots of wildflowers in season, Ward Creek nearby, and wonderful views of the Sierra Crest above.

For more information about hiking and backpacking with children, pick up a copy of my book *Monsters in the Woods: Backpacking with Children,* published by the University of Nevada Press.

What About Fido?

While dogs are allowed on much of the Tahoe Rim Trail, restrictions do apply at several state parks, including Lake Tahoe Nevada State Park. In fact, regulations governing dogs on trails completely depend on what county you are passing through. It is your responsibility to know what the specific regulations are under each county's jurisdiction. In general, it is best to leave the

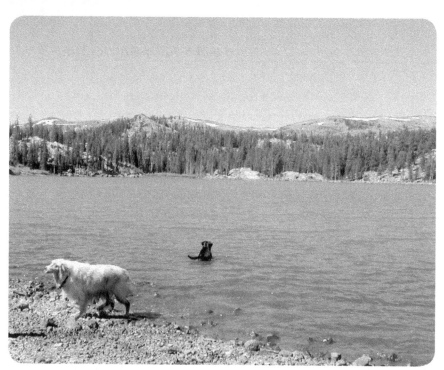
Dogs love Round Lake.

pups at home or at least keep them on a leash. Off-leash dogs chase and interfere with wildlife and trample the understory of forests. Your chances of encountering wild creatures will increase, and you'll have the satisfaction of knowing that you are limiting your effect on the trail. If you do hike with your pooch, be sure to have him or her on a leash or under voice command at all times. Dogs jumping on other hikers, chasing mountain bikers, running beyond your sight line, or harassing horses are a big no-no. If you have a well trained, on-leash animal that doesn't go after every squirrel or chase every lizard, by all means take him or her along.

6

Trail Description

These trail descriptions list point-to-point mileages. The mileage figures are based on several sources; the primary sources for the maps you see in this book are Tom Harrison's *Lake Tahoe Recreation Map,* which has been enhanced with information generously provided by Jeffrey P. Schaffer, whose *Tahoe Sierra* and *Pacific Crest Trail: Northern California* set the standard for guidebooks in this area. These figures give you distances between certain locations. However, you should realize that when it says 0.9 mile, another source might report it as 1.1 miles. If this difference really bothers you, perhaps you need to relax a bit. I have found the best way to relax is to spend time walking in the woods. For your convenience, a mileage chart for the Tahoe Rim Trail appears in Appendix A (page 208).

Before each description, I recommend when the section can be hiked without encountering large amounts of snow. These dates are estimates based on an "average snow year," but there is no such thing as an *average* year. It either snows more than average or less than average. The dates should give you a rough idea of when you can hike. If it has been an especially mild winter and a warm spring, you could expect to hike the trail sooner than the dates stated here. Refer to Chapter 4 (page 36) on weather for more detail about snow seasons.

Finally, the Tahoe Rim Trail is constantly evolving. Minor trail changes for maintenance and realignment are being planned and implemented on a regular basis. Although this book attempts to be up-to-date, changes to the trail may have been made since this book was published. For more information about any recent changes to the trail, contact the Tahoe Rim Trail Association at (775) 298-0012.

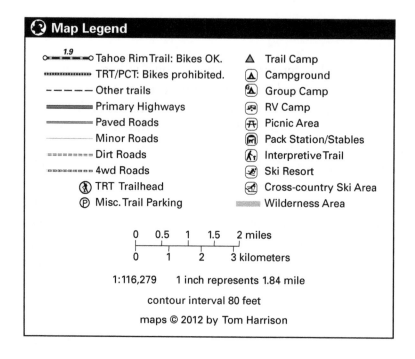

Map Legend

○━ ━ ━ ━○ Tahoe Rim Trail: Bikes OK.	▲ Trail Camp
▪▪▪▪▪▪▪▪▪▪▪ TRT/PCT: Bikes prohibited.	Ⓐ Campground
─ ─ ─ ─ ─ Other trails	Group Camp
━━━━━ Primary Highways	RV Camp
━━━━ Paved Roads	Picnic Area
──── Minor Roads	Pack Station/Stables
════════ Dirt Roads	Interpretive Trail
▫▫▫▫▫▫▫▫ 4wd Roads	Ski Resort
Ⓧ TRT Trailhead	Cross-country Ski Area
Ⓟ Misc. Trail Parking	▬▬▬ Wilderness Area

0   0.5   1   1.5   2 miles

0   1   2   3 kilometers

1:116,279   1 inch represents 1.84 mile

contour interval 80 feet

maps © 2012 by Tom Harrison

Tahoe City to Brockway Summit
(20.2 miles)

Difficulty This section is strenuous. It is long, requires a good deal of climbing, and can be quite hot in the summer when it is also mostly waterless.

Best Seasons While portions of the trail at lower elevations are accessible from late May to early November, higher elevation areas have snow until later. The snow melts first along the first several miles north of Tahoe City.

Highlights This section includes a several-mile jaunt along the edge of the Truckee River Canyon with excellent views of Lake Tahoe and the Truckee River. Much of the area has been logged extensively over the years, so you will see mostly smaller, newer growth trees and a wide variety of species as you move through the different elevations. The section above the Truckee River has several incredible sugar pine and Jeffrey pine specimens. The trail has outstanding views of Alpine Meadows and Squaw Valley. Watson Lake, while not the most beautiful lake along the Tahoe Rim Trail, is a pleasant shallow lake nestled among the trees two-thirds of the way through your hike.

Heads Up! This is a long stretch, and water is in short supply. Year-round water sources do not exist, except for Watson Lake, which is 13.4 miles from Tahoe City and 6.7 miles from Brockway Summit. Watson Lake is shallow, and its water looks unenticing to drink. (These days, you should treat water from even the most sparkling lakes.) A stream east of Watson Lake may be available in the early season. Bring lots of water if you're hiking this section! With many road crossings and much off-highway-vehicle (OHV) use, don't be surprised to hear or see cars close to the trail. Watson Lake can be accessed via a paved road and is heavily used by car campers and occasionally by late night partiers. For

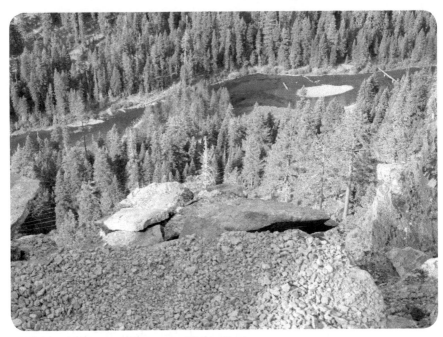
Truckee River from the TRT north of Tahoe City

mountain bikers, the rocky terrain can be challenging, even frustrating. This section is not recommended for beginner riders. If you hiked the first 5 miles out of Tahoe City before the reroute of 2007 and were pleasantly surprised to see a dearth of mountain bikes, those days are over—the reroute has made that section a popular place to ride.

Getting There, Tahoe City to Brockway From the Tahoe City "Y" at the intersection of Highways 89 and 28, go 0.2 mile west on Highway 89 toward Truckee. Just past a gas station (a Chevron at the time this book is published), turn right on Fairway Drive. Drive another 0.2 mile to a parking lot and the Fairway Community Center on the right. If this parking lot is full, you can park (on weekends only) at the Tahoe City Public Utility District offices about 0.1 mile back toward Highway 89. Your trailhead is across the street from the center.

Getting There, Brockway to Tahoe City From the intersection of Highway 28 and Highway 267 in Kings Beach, drive 2.75 miles north on Highway 267 to the TRT trailhead. Look carefully—it is easy to miss. Parking is available at the road pullout on the left, 0.5 mile before Brockway Summit. The trail starts at the downhill edge of the parking area. If you plan on mountain biking this section, it is best to head south from Brockway Summit toward Tahoe City, although either direction will challenge you with steep, rocky terrain that includes technically challenging sections.

Trail Description

From the Tahoe City Trailhead, the trail starts out as a moderate 10-percent uphill grade and passes through thick sections of manzanita, patches of squaw carpet, and a forest of white fir, Jeffrey pine, sugar pine, and incense cedar trees. Several views of Tahoe City and the lake open up beyond. After about 0.7 mile you cross a dirt road; for a little history lesson, detour right and climb steeply uphill about 100 yards and then turn right. You will see a white cross that sits above Tahoe City (see side trip "Boyle's Last Ride").

Back on the Tahoe Rim Trail, you quickly reach a hard-to-locate junction, where the old TRT has been decommissioned. In 2007 4 miles of trail were relocated farther to the west and along the Truckee River Canyon. If you hiked this trail before 2007 you are in for a treat. The views and walking tread on the new section are dramatically better than that of the old trail. Shortly, you make the first of many crossings of what locals call the Fiberboard Freeway (also Road 16N73 or Forest Route 73), after the company that was once the principal landholder in the area. The term *freeway* is derived from the fact that while at this point it is a nar-

SIDE TRIP Boyle's Last Ride

According to local legend, William Boyle was an easy-going codger with a dry sense of humor who lived in Tahoe City in the early 20th century. He once asked his drinking buddies to bury him above the town so he could keep an eye on them. True to their word, when he died, his friends dragged Boyle's body up the hill on a sled and buried him above Tahoe City on February 4, 1912. Shortly afterward, the cross was erected at the site. Photos taken at that time period show a clear, treeless view down to the lake. Now, however, trees and brush have grown so thickly that much of the view from the cross has been obscured.

Lake Tahoe from Tahoe Cross-Country Ski Area

row dirt road, later in our hike it becomes a wide gravel road and the main backcountry route linking Tahoe City and Brockway Summit (and via another connection, Truckee). After crossing the road, you quickly reach a seasonal stream, before a small climb to your first major lake view. Here in addition to a healthy swath of Lake Tahoe you see the Granlibakken ski area and its surrounding neighborhood. For folks in Tahoe City looking for quick access to a great view, you can hike to this view and back to your trailhead in less than an hour.

While you have been heading west, now the trail heads north, following the ridgetop of the Truckee River Canyon for the next 4 miles. The ascent is steady, but not overly strenuous, and the views are some of the most unique on the entire Tahoe Rim Trail. After a saunter along the ridgeline, the trail takes a brief foray into a thick forest of white fir, where you may find some of the biggest pinedrops you will ever encounter. Soon enough, you are back on the canyon edge, marveling at the majestic sugar pines and Jeffrey pines as you meander along the lava-topped ridge. After another section of climbing through thicker forest, you gently descend to an open field of green, a seasonal creek crossing, and a short climb

Pacific Crest from the Tahoe Rim Trail north of Tahoe City

at about 3 miles from the trailhead to a stunning viewpoint: A cliff's edge lava flat bordered by gnarled junipers overlooking the Truckee River below, where summertime rafters can be heard and seen. If you can look up from the river view, Twin Peaks looks pretty impressive as well.

The good stuff continues for the next half mile as the trail follows the ridge with views of Squaw and Alpine a constant companion. Alas, all things must come to an end, and you leave the ridgeline and head into the forest for a sustained mile-plus climb. Your trail switchbacks through sections of thicker forest and recently thinned sections before passing waves of pinemat manzanita where the forest canopy changes from white to red fir.

A last traverse brings you to nifty trail work through a pile of volcanic rocks and the first of two awesome lunch spots, both with plenty of rocks to sit on to enjoy the views. This first vista includes Lake Tahoe, Twin Peaks, and parts of Alpine Meadows. The next one, just 200 yards farther, looks directly into the entrance to Alpine Meadows and a good portion of Squaw Valley. The second view sits on a big pile of fractured basalt; when you walk over it, it sounds like broken glass, which apparently is enough for many mountain bikers to refer to this popular section of trail as "Glass Mountain."

Next the trail follows the ridge and you soon see to your right, the dark red volcanic rock of the Cinder Cone. Longtime Tahoe locals will tell you that this cinder cone area was the repository for Tahoe City sewer water before the treatment plant was built in Truckee in the 1970s. Does that change your mind about where you planned to stop for lunch? As the trail skirts the Cinder Cone you see the remnants of an old fence. (See side trip "Cinder Cone.")

Past the Cinder Cone the trail heads north for 0.5 mile and then descends rather steeply through a small north-facing section of thick forest (which will hold snow into summer) to an open saddle at the end of a little-used dirt road. Here you begin heading gently uphill through an open forest of fir trees and manzanita. Quickly the trail proceeds downhill again, and the forest becomes thicker and your hike, shadier.

> **SIDE TRIP Cinder Cone**
>
> Leave the trail and walk east onto the mostly flat, red surface of the Cinder Cone. The lack of plant growth and evidence of filled-in ditches clearly show that the site was once affected by human use. It has been a long time, however, since this area was used for water treatment, and it is recovering nicely.

Like most of the northern and western shores of Lake Tahoe, this area has been logged heavily in the past. The most extensive logging occurred in the late 1800s when much of the Tahoe Basin was logged to make braces in the silver mines of nearby Virginia City to keep them from collapsing (as well as for lumber and fuel). Loggers at that time focused on the best trees for their purposes—the pine trees, especially the majestic sugar pine—and left most of the fir trees. During an extended wet period, the red and white firs took over the territory from the more drought- and disease-resistant Jeffrey and sugar pines, creating an unnaturally dense forest made up primarily of firs. If nature had been allowed to revert to its own natural process, periodic forest fires would

SIDE TRIP "The Wall"

A left turn here would quickly take you 300 yards northwest to a minor saddle and the start of a steep downhill, known as "The Wall" by mountain biking enthusiasts. It leads to the Western States Trail and in a few steep downhill miles to the bike trail at the bridge across the Truckee River between Squaw Valley and Alpine Meadows. The bike trail leads back to Tahoe City and the beginning of the TRT; it makes a nice loop for experienced bikers.

have thinned the population of fir. Instead, the federal and state governments, under heavy pressure to prevent forest fires and to limit tree cutting, had a policy of preventing major forest fires by putting out all fires as quickly as possible. In the short-term this policy saved the forest, but it led to a denser forest and increased the likelihood of a catastrophic fire. We now know that this historic policy excluded the ecological role of frequent natural fires. Expansive stands of dead trees in an overly thick forest are a recipe for disaster. The National Forest Service and both the Nevada and California State Park Departments have begun an aggressive effort of salvage logging and controlled burning to reduce the danger. As you walk or ride on the Tahoe Rim Trail, you may see evidence of this effort in the form of brush piles waiting to be burned and stumps from recent logging in many locations.

About 1 mile past the last dirt road, you cross another dirt road (see side trip "The Wall"). This one is in a dry gully above the headwaters of Burton Creek. Those desperate for water can head 0.75 mile southeast down the road to its end at the Fiberboard Freeway (Forest Route 73). Turn left there, and head briefly north to the creek, which may dry up after a mild winter.

To continue on the TRT, cross this second dirt road to enter prime mountain biking terrain. The amount of trail traffic will increase dramatically. The trail here is part of a network of trails providing great biking opportunities out of Tahoe City and the Tahoe Cross-Country Ski Area located in the Highlands subdivision. The next stage is a mostly moderate climb through soft volcanic dirt and mixed forest 0.9 mile to the east edge of Painted Rock (7754 feet). Along the way you pass some impressive volcanic boulders. After the climb to Painted Rock, you're rewarded with two good viewpoints: One offers a panorama southeast toward Lake Tahoe; another spot a little farther gives you an awe-inspiring view into Squaw Valley backed by the Sierra Crest.

After all the uphill work you have done in the last 8 miles, you get a break with a mostly shady descent (or if on a bike, a really fun downhill) to another crossing of the Fiberboard Freeway at about 9 miles from the Tahoe City Trailhead. Here, usually on the first Sunday in March, the Great Ski Race passes this point on its way to Truckee. This 30-kilometer cross-country ski race, from the Tahoe Cross-Country Ski Area on Dollar Hill to Truckee, attracts up to a thousand people, making it one of the biggest cross-country ski events in the western United States. For the next 0.8 mile you cover a smooth, gentle incline over hard-packed sandy soils (mountain bikers should ride it back down to enjoy one of the best biking stretches on the whole TRT). Where the trail levels off and runs into an old narrow dirt road, a left turn will take you 100 yards north to the Fiberboard Freeway (see side trip "Mount Watson").

Just south of the Fiberboard Freeway, take the TRT; it turns right and follows an old abandoned dirt road, now overgrown with manzanita and tobacco brush. This gentle downhill stretch continues 1.6 miles, providing several excellent lake views

SIDE TRIP Mount Watson

A left turn at the Fiberboard Freeway will take you back to Tahoe City, while a right turn will take you to Truckee, Brockway Summit, or to the top of Mt. Watson. Should you want to climb or ride to Mt. Watson, follow the freeway uphill from where it meets the dirt road for 0.7 mile to a junction with a major dirt road that turns sharply right (southeast). Turn onto this road, and follow it for 1 mile on a 640-foot ascent to the top of Mt. Watson (8424 feet). Views from the top are glorious; you can see most of Lake Tahoe and its surrounding mountains as well as Squaw Valley and Alpine Meadows to the west.

before a left turn heads you back uphill. You now wind uphill, northeast, between lava boulders and cliffs for the next 0.75 mile to a wonderful stopping place among several especially large boulders, with enticing views of the lake to the south between

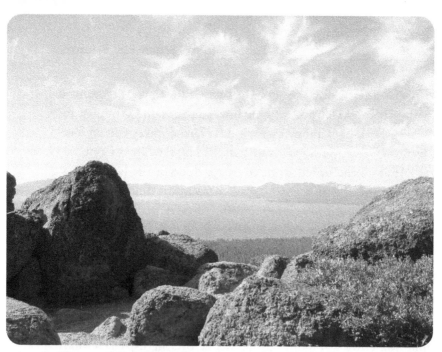
Lava boulders near Watson Lake

the boulders. That large white-roofed building in the foreground is my alma mater, North Tahoe High School. Beyond the viewpoint, the trail levels off and turns right before it reaches another junction, 1 mile short of Watson Lake. (A left turn here would take you steeply uphill to the top of Mt. Watson.)

Continue straight ahead on the TRT on a moderately steep downhill toward Watson Lake. Just before the lake, you reach a gravel road; turn left on this road and follow it uphill. In a short distance, the TRT takes off to the right and skirts the east shore of Watson Lake. While little Watson Lake is pleasant enough, it is shallow, surrounded by trees, and visited by numerous mosquitoes. It can also be heavily used in the summer since it is the only lake between Brockway Summit and Tahoe City and accessible by car along a paved and gravel road. Be sure to filter any water you get from Watson Lake.

After you pass the lake, with 13.4 miles under your belt and 6.7 miles to go, the TRT heads about 0.25 mile north to a shallow gully. The trail now descends gently 1.25 miles east through beautiful wildflower meadows and forested areas, to a road, down which you can head 0.3 mile to usually reliable Watson Creek. You pass several small seep streams that provide water until mid-summer. Since these are the last water sources along this section, take advantage of the opportunity if it's still available. Just 0.25 mile east beyond the road, a short (90 yards) spur trail leads off to the right to a large rock pile with another pretty view of Lake Tahoe, specifically Carnelian Bay. Enjoy the view—it's the last full lake view you get before you reach the Brockway Summit Trailhead in about 4.5 miles.

The trail turns north and in 0.8 mile switchbacks down through a thick forest of white fir and Jeffrey pine to a crossing of Forest Route 74, and 100 yards farther crosses Forest Route 75. After a gentle descent northeast for about two-thirds of a mile, you cross another road, then traverse about 200 yards to yet another. Now you have a fairly gentle climb for 1 mile as the trail takes you through manzanita and chinquapin before it crosses Forest Service Road 73 (Fiberboard Freeway). There is still more climbing for 1.3 miles until you cross the Fiberboard Freeway one more time. The next 0.7 mile gently descends to the trailhead, located next to Highway 267. At this point, you are about 0.5 mile east of Brockway Summit.

Brockway Summit to Mount Rose Trailhead

(20.2 miles)

Difficulty With much of this section of the trail rising above 9000 feet and some of it higher than 10,000 feet in elevation, it is relatively strenuous, especially considering that you start at around 7000 feet. If you are dayhiking this section, it might be easier to begin on the Tahoe Meadows side and hike to Brockway Summit, where your starting elevation is approximately 8800 feet. As they say, 1800 feet here and 1800 feet there and eventually you are talking about some real elevation gain.

Best Seasons The entire trail can be hiked between late July and mid-October. The first 5 miles from the Brockway end can be hiked as early as June, but most of the trail is not free of snow until mid-July. The highest sections of the trail are among the first places to be covered with snow in the fall.

Highlights The middle part of this trail section is mostly exposed, south-facing volcanic slopes with sandy soils. This wide expanse at a high altitude features tremendous panoramic views of the lake and a wonderful feeling of remoteness. Two small lakes are found on the trail or close to it: small Mud Lake and Gray Lake, a prettier, knee-deep lake that is 0.5 mile off the Rim Trail via an access trail. A lovely waterfall, several streams, awesome high altitude views, and prolific wildflower displays await you along the last 6 miles of your route.

Heads Up! Since much of this hike is at high altitude, the air is quite thin, which can cause problems for those unaccustomed to high altitudes. If you feel faint, it may be because of reduced oxygen levels rather than the beauty of the views. Much of the trail is exposed to cold and wind or to the hot sun. The first 5 miles can

Mount Houghton from the new section of the TRT near Mount Rose

be tedious, but the remainder is a wonderful high-altitude experience. Though you can collect water from several seasonal streams, as well as from Gray Lake and usually from Mud Lake, the supply is severely limited. A small seasonal spring exists about 50 feet below where the TRT meets the old Western States Trail and Incline Lake Trail after Mud Lake. Gray Lake is about 0.9 mile downhill from a saddle just past Mud Lake, and Mud Lake itself lives up to its name by becoming a mud puddle by late summer. About 2.5 miles from the end of the trail, you'll find water cascading down from Galena Falls.

Tips for Mountain Bikers If you are looking for a good section of the Tahoe Rim Trail to ride, this is probably not the one to choose. Please do not ride on the portion of this trail that does *not* allow bikes! The soil on that stretch is quite fragile and easily damaged.

From the Brockway Summit side, bikes are allowed for the first 7.6 miles. It begins with a steady, technical, and sometimes steep climb of 4.3 miles to a major gravel road. From here you can take a left turn and head back to the highway on the road.

On the way back to the highway, you will pass Martis Peak Rd., which heads up to the Martis Peak Fire Lookout, with spectacular views to the north. Back on the TRT you could turn right and ride another mile, but it gets even steeper and more technical and may not be worth the effort.

The TRT from the Mt. Rose Summit Trailhead has two alternate routes. The first parallels Highway 431, 0.5 mile to a dirt road, where you turn right and ride 2.1 miles to the Snow Pond. This route allows mountain bikers and horses. The second route, which begins to the right and above the bike route, allows only hikers. From Snow Pond it is a moderately steep and rocky uphill for 1.5 miles on dirt road to the radio tower, which is the end of the trail for bikers.

Getting There, Brockway to Mt. Rose Summit Trailhead (Tahoe Meadows) From the intersection of Highways 28 and 267 in Kings Beach, drive 2.75 miles northwest up Highway 267 toward Brockway Summit to the Tahoe Rim Trail Trailhead. At this point, you will see a parking pullout on the left and a steep dirt road on the right (Forest Service Road 16N56). Park on either side, but this trailhead is on the right (uphill) side. If you reach Brockway Summit at the top of the hill, you have gone 0.5 mile too far.

Getting There, Mt. Rose Summit Trailhead to Brockway Take Highway 431 (Mt. Rose Highway) to Tahoe Meadows and then on to the trailhead just at the summit of the Mt. Rose Highway. The Mt. Rose Trailhead is 8 miles from the intersection of Highways 431 and 28 in Incline Village, and 0.7 mile from the Tahoe Meadows South Trailhead. It is directly across the highway from Mt. Rose Campground, which can be a great camping spot for thru-hikers or a way station the night before you begin your TRT hike.

Alternative Routes A trail that will be known as the Rim to Reno Trail is currently under construction; it will allow hikers to travel from the outskirts of Reno through the Mt. Rose Wilderness to the Mt. Rose Trail and the Mt. Rose Trailhead.

Trail Description

From the Brockway Trailhead, cross the busy road carefully if you are parked on the south side of Highway 267, and follow the dirt road uphill (east) 100 yards to the trail and trailhead sign. The trail leads off to the left into the trees. This first section is no-nonsense, fairly steep, with occasional views of the lake as you switchback through a thick forest of newer growth Jeffrey pines and white firs. Walk quickly to escape the drone of automobile traffic from the road below. After about 0.5 mile, the views get better as you pass through an area of manzanita and squaw carpet. In early summer you will also encounter numerous wildflowers. Listen closely and you may hear the mating call of a blue grouse; it sounds like a bass drum, "*brmmmmm, brmmmmm, brmmmmm.*"

After about 1 mile of steady climbing, you reach a junction at 1.2 miles from the trailhead (see side trip "View from a Rock").

The TRT continues straight ahead on a ridge, descending briefly before leveling off. Here it becomes more open; you will see fewer trees in a more scattered pattern, along with mules ears, a very common plant with large leaves and large yellow flowers. About 0.7 mile past the spur trail, you cross a gravel road (16N33) about 150 yards east of its junction with paved Martis Peak Road. You start heading up again gently and then go downhill briefly to a small grassy opening with early summer flowers and a streamlet providing water in the springtime.

Next, head steeply up again through a forest that is transitioning from Jeffrey pines and white firs to the higher-altitude lodge-

SIDE TRIP **View from a Rock**

On your left is a short spur trail, which heads 0.3 mile up to a pile of rocks that look as though it was part of a set for *The Flintstones*. From atop the rocks, you get great lake views to the south and mountain views to the north and west. This is a very popular summertime spot to catch the last rays of the sun, and if you are camping, a good spot to see the sunrise.

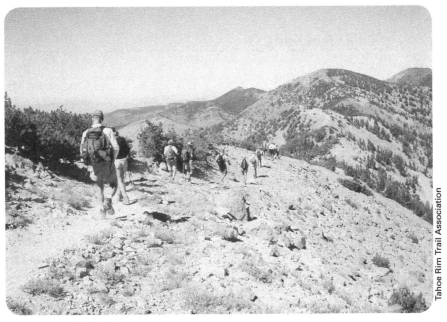

Hikers near Relay Peak

pole pines and red firs. The air is thick with the pungent cinnamon aroma of tobacco brush. Your climb eases, and you come out of the forest into a huge field of equally aromatic mules ears. Continuing uphill you leave the thick forest and the scenery changes dramatically. You reach an open rock pile, almost 4 miles from the trailhead that hosts dramatic views to the south of Lake Tahoe. Looking to the south across the lake, you can see (clockwise from east to west) Snow Valley Peak (9914 feet), the highest peak above the east shore; Jobs Sister (10,823 feet); Freel Peak (10,881 feet); South Lake Tahoe; Mt. Tallac (9735 feet); Desolation Wilderness and the Crystal Range; Twin Peaks (8878 feet) above the west shore; and finally Squaw Valley and Northstar. Freel Peak and Jobs Sister are the two highest peaks in the Tahoe Basin. If you continue on the TRT for another 70 miles you will walk just below Freel Peak as you cross a saddle at 9730 feet. If you enjoy sitting in the sunshine while eating your lunch, this south-facing spot may be just the ticket. On September 22, 2001, this viewpoint was the location for the official opening dedication ceremony for the TRT.

When you can drag yourself away from the panoramic views of the lake, continue up rocky terrain along the edge of a ridge.

SIDE TRIP **Martis Peak Lookout**

A left turn on this dirt road takes you to the Martis Peak (8742 feet) lookout. To get there go 0.2 mile and then turn right and take the paved road 0.7 mile up to the lookout at 8656 feet. From here you will see excellent views of most of Lake Tahoe and the crest that rims it to the south, and to the north, most of the lands from the Donner Pass and Lake environs east into western Nevada.

You will have a clear view of Mt. Baldy to the east and the beautiful aspen groves along its flanks. With Mt. Baldy as your goal, you pass a rocky viewpoint to your right and a field full of mules ears to your left, before heading back into the woods again briefly and reaching a major dirt road at 4.3 miles in from your trailhead (see side trip "Martis Peak Lookout").

This dirt road makes a good alternative trailhead for those who would like to hike 16, instead of 20, miles. Since it sits at 8400 feet you can also eliminate 1400 feet of climbing by beginning here. To access the dirt road, turn on Martis Peak Road, which is about 0.5 mile north of Brockway Summit. Follow this paved road as it climbs up and up, and at a big left turn 4 miles in, the dirt road heads straight ahead. Go about 0.2 mile to the trailhead on your right.

The TRT turns to the right and follows the dusty road about 0.25 mile north to a fork. Keep left and gently ascend 300 yards north to a trailhead with parking for several vehicles. You have now reached a part of the old Western States Trail, also known as the Capital-to-Capital Trail because it once linked Carson City (the capital of Nevada) with Sacramento (the capital of California). The trail starts east through forest and alternating open rocky sections and in 0.5 mile reaches a saddle with views north. The tree composition is transitioning again with more red firs and occasional junipers, western white pines, and the first hemlocks that you see on this section. Your climb becomes steeper as you switchback 0.3 mile up to a ridgeline that has views into a large U-shaped valley, the drainage area for Juniper Creek, which empties into the Truckee River.

Above Tahoe Meadows

After about a 300-yard traverse southeast on the ridgeline, the trail angles south for a 0.4-mile traverse of gentle slopes to a road; from here, the trail ascends 0.2 mile south to the road's end and the resumption of trail tread. In less than 0.5 mile you climb first moderately southeast and then moderately northeast up to the ridgeline. There's a great view here, but even more superlative ones lie ahead. Just 0.2 mile south you reach a low rock pile immediately west of the trail, which has dramatic views of the lake to the south and of the mountains to the west and east. In addition, there are great views to the north; you can see Castle Peak, Donner Lake, the town of Truckee, and Boca and Stampede Reservoirs.

From this view, you are now about 6.8 miles from the Brockway Summit Trailhead. The TRT goes briefly east to the ridgeline, where you cross into Nevada. (This is a good place to turn around if you are on a bike.) As the trees get smaller and fewer, and you get higher, now above 9000 feet, the ridgeline area opens up. Only the hardiest trees, such as lodgepole, western white, and whitebark pine grow here. On the north-facing slopes below and also east of you, snow may last well into the summer.

After climbing moderately southeast 0.5 mile up the ridgeline, the TRT angles northeast, traversing just under a minor summit on a high ridge, which is 9271-foot Mt. Baldy. Just past it, you enter the Mt. Rose Wilderness. At about 7.6 miles from the trailhead, this is the end of the section of trail permissible to mountain bikes. Bike riding is not allowed in the wilderness. (A better place to turn around is the viewpoint you just passed or where the trail met the dirt road, 4.3 miles from the Brockway Trailhead.)

Now you traverse the side of an open southeast-facing slope with incredible expansive views to the south and east of Lake Tahoe, Incline Village, and beyond. For the next 2 miles, with the exception of a brief uphill foray into the forest, you walk beneath a volcanic ridge eastward on a gentle ascent over wonderful light brown, sandy soil through huge open fields of mules ears. Views of the lake are truly glorious with almost the entire lake displayed before you. It is a real highlight of the Tahoe Rim Trail, and considering how far you are from either the Tahoe Meadows or Brockway Trailheads, you may even have it all to yourself.

About midway on your northeast traverse you pass just beneath a steep-sided 9499-foot summit, behind which lies unseen, flat-topped Rifle Peak. In 0.5 mile you traverse beneath pyramidal Rose Knob, and then in another 0.7 mile reach a junction. At about 10 miles from the Brockway Summit Trailhead, you have reached the new access trail to Gray Lake (see side trip "Gray Lake").

From its first junction with the Gray Lake Trail, the TRT stays high and continues straight ahead, east across south-facing slopes toward Rose Knob Peak (9710 feet), an impressive pile of volcanic rock with three distinct pointy peaks. After a 0.5-mile traverse across slopes, the TRT crosses a saddle with clusters of whitebark pines and then soon climbs 0.25 mile southeast, where it passes beneath the southernmost summit of Rose Knob Peak. Then the trail rounds the bend and travels northeast across talus on the south-facing side of the mountain.

This rocky section was one of the last parts of the trail to be completed, and one of the most difficult to build. The trail build-

SIDE TRIP Gray Lake

While the old Gray Lake Trail began on a steep, north-facing, potentially dangerous slope, the new trail built in 2011 starts out on a level section of ridge and descends gently through a grove of hemlocks—great job, trailbuilders. It then makes a meandering, moderate descent 0.6 mile northeast down to clear, but knee-deep Gray Lake, where a new loop trail around the lake provides access to excellent campsites above its north shore. A beautiful mountain stream leads past lush wildflowers into the lake from the huge rock fall below Rose Knob Peak and then drains out of the lake near the lake's biggest campsite.

While in early and midsummer the lake can be a haven for mosquitoes, in the fall it is a pleasant and quiet place to relax. At 9043 feet this lake with marshy surroundings is quite fragile; take extra care to not damage the plants near the lake. Note the especially large lodgepole and whitebark pines and hemlocks in this idyllic setting. Also of note, with its very shallow depth and location in a high-altitude bowl, Gray Lake sometimes has ice on its surface well before you would see ice anywhere else—one time on a cold August morning. As the only dependable lake between Watson Lake and Star Lake, Gray Lake is well worth a stop.

From Gray Lake a rebuilt trail takes you back to an intersection with the TRT above Mud Lake. The former very steep 0.5-mile trail, has been replaced by a well-laid-out 0.9-mile climb that takes full advantage of the views. Why not visit Mud Lake, which is just below us to the right from the Gray Lake trail junction with the TRT? Here's why: Mud Lake lives up to its name. In late summer it gets quite small before sometimes disappearing altogether.

ers have constructed formidable rock walls and created a fairly smooth trail through the talus field. As you go around the mountain you once again enjoy magnificent views of almost the entire lake. After a 0.3-mile traverse mostly across talus, the trail angles north and contours over to a saddle above Mud Lake; this stretch has a few scattered mountain hemlocks. At the east edge of the saddle is a junction with the Gray Lake Trail, about 11.2 miles from the Brockway Summit Trailhead and 9 miles from the Mt. Rose Trailhead.

From the saddle between Mud Lake and Gray Lake, the Tahoe Rim Trail goes right (southeast) and descends gently 0.25 mile on an open slope above Mud Lake, with additional spectacular views all the way to Fallen Leaf Lake at the far end of Lake Tahoe, in the distance to the south. The TRT then traverses 0.25 mile northeast,

SIDE TRIP Incline Lake Trail

Until recently, Incline Lake was a small lake visible from the old TRT (road) to Snow Pond that headed up from Tahoe Meadows. Access into the area of private homes, however, was prohibited. And more importantly, access to this trail, which in just 2 miles goes from Tahoe Meadows to the Tahoe Rim Trail near Gray Lake, was private as well. Now the Forest Service owns the land, which opens up lots of wonderful opportunities for hiking in the area.

The Incline Lake Trailhead is on the north side of Highway 431, across the busy highway from the Ophir Creek Trail, right at the edge of Tahoe Meadows. You begin by walking past the gate to an aspen-lined, paved road, which in a half mile leads to a big left turn where the trail begins with a short downhill to a creek crossing. Then a 1.5-mile ascent begins. While the trail is quite steep at times, you walk through some of the largest ancient western white pines, hemlocks, and lodgepoles that I have seen. In the last half mile you cross another stream, pass the Mt. Rose Wilderness boundary, and reach a saddle with great views of Lake Tahoe. A short easy descent brings you to the TRT at its low point between Mud Lake and Relay Peak.

Via the Incline Lake Trail, you can hike to Gray Lake, loop around Rose Knob Peak, and return to your car at Tahoe Meadows in just 8 miles. You can also turn right where the Incline Lake Trail meets the TRT, climb up to Relay Peak, follow the trail past the waterfall to the Mt. Rose Trailhead, and then cross Tahoe Meadows back to the Incline Lake Trailhead. This 12-mile loop provides a tremendous amount of hiking bang for your buck.

exchanging volcanic treaad for granite (to be followed shortly by more volcanic tread briefly before returning to granite). You reach a junction with the Incline Lake Trail and former Western States Trail (see side trip "Incline Lake Trail").

About 50 feet below this junction, near some willows, is a small spring that can provide water for most of the season. After the snow melts, this is your last source for water until you get to Galena Falls about 6 miles away. You could also head downhill steeply about a half mile for water on the Incline Lake Trail.

With about 8 miles remaining, start up the TRT on a series of short switchbacks. You soon traverse just below a dramatic large red-and-black volcanic rock at the top of a ridge. The trail passes just below and to the east of this rock and climbs slightly to the north-facing side of the mountain about 0.75 mile past the junction. Below is Ginny Lake, and in the distance are Tahoe

Tamarack Peak

Meadows, the Mt. Rose Highway, and Mt. Rose itself. You now traverse slightly uphill across the north-facing slope to a saddle just below a granite ridge. Here you have crossed a steep slope that is covered in snow most of the year—take care if the pathway is icy. The terrain is spectacular with several large craggy volcanic rocks towering above and a hemlock forest below.

At the saddle, you now face your second 800-foot climb; the first was up to the wilderness boundary below Mt. Baldy. The imposing massif straight ahead would be formidable if you tackled it head-on, but fortunately the TRT does not, and the climb is exceptionally well-graded. From the saddle the TRT has several short switchbacks up among granite boulders, and then it jogs east, then west. Here, it climbs 0.6 mile north with abundant views to a switchback just above the east end of a west-trending ridge that climbs to the summit of Relay Peak. Along this ascent, Clark's nutcrackers flit between the scattered gnarled whitebark and western white pines.

From the switchback, huge panoramic views open up to the west of Castle Peak, Donner Lake, and the Truckee area and to the south in the distance of Freel Peak above Lake Tahoe. From

Rock pile near the California-Nevada border above Lake Tahoe

your vantage point you also have closer views: west down the gaping West Fork Gray Creek Canyon, a close-up of the nearby Slab Cliffs, northwest down equally gaping Gray Creek Canyon, and northeast to a radio-towered peak.

From this switchback, where snow can linger well into July, you are about halfway up your major ascent. The TRT climbs 0.5 mile southeast up volcanic slopes, and you surpass 10,000 feet in elevation before you reach a switchback that has poor views. You now have two shorter switchback legs to Relay Peak, the highest point on the entire Tahoe Rim Trail at 10,338 feet in elevation. On a clear day you can see all the way to Lassen Peak and, rumor has it, Mt. Shasta if the day is crystal clear. The panorama seems unlimited as dozens of narrow valleys and ridgelines unfold before you. Much of what you see in the foreground is the Mt. Rose Wilderness. Mt. Rose (10,776 feet) itself stands out to the northeast in its full volcanic relief. At sunset, the mountain certainly lives up to its name as it takes on a beautiful rosy hue. To the east-southeast, beyond Tahoe Meadows and the Ophir Creek Canyon, lies large Washoe Lake.

From Relay Peak your trail now merges with an abandoned dirt road that heads downhill steeply north along the ridgeline

Looking southwest toward Dollar Point and the Pacific Crest

to a relay microwave tower developed by AT&T. While the top of the ridgeline provides an excellent location for receiving radio waves, it is unfortunate to see a large ugly tower in this incredibly beautiful location. Near the tower you reach a junction with a broad gravel road, which is still used by vehicles for administrative purposes. Over the next 5 miles you will encounter a number of junctions and trail options. The good news is that recent trail building in the area has provided some great options for loops in the Mt. Rose and Tahoe Meadows area. The bad news is that it may be a bit of a challenge to keep track of it all. Listen closely and use a map.

Old TRT: If you turn right on this broad utility road you will be on the old Tahoe Rim Trail and the section that allows bikes. First you descend 0.3 mile south to a switchback and then 0.5 mile northward to a bend east, where you pass an old equipment lift. Before the road to the top of the ridge was built, this lift was constructed as a means to bring the building materials necessary for the relay tower to the top of the mountain; later the lift was used to access the tower during extreme winter periods when snowcats were unable

Mount Rose from Relay Peak

to make the trip to the top. The road descends into a big open bowl with scattered stunted whitebark pine trees. In the winter this area is popular with skiers, snowshoers, and snowmobilers.

Now after 1.4 miles of moderately steep downhill on the road, you reach a small pond, known both as Snow Pond (because it is covered in snow much of the year) and as Frog Pond. About 1 mile past the pond you get full views of Incline Lake, Lake Tahoe, and Tahoe Meadows. Far below, the next section of the TRT can look like a brown snake wandering through the deep green of Tahoe Meadows. The views remain panoramic and inspiring as the road continues gently downhill to a junction with a single-track trail at about 2.1 miles from the Snow Pond. Here the trail turns left and traverses gently uphill to the Mt. Rose Summit Trailhead. (If you stay on the dirt road straight ahead you will quickly reach Highway 431, where you can turn left and go 0.3 mile to the Mt. Rose Summit Trailhead, or turn right and go 0.4 mile to the Tahoe Meadows Trailhead.)

New TRT: The new TRT, which was still under construction when I wrote this description for the third edition, follows the ridgeline to the north of the Relay Tower and then along the gentle ridge down to a saddle. You pass scattered whitebark pines and are treated to breathtaking views of Snow Pond, Slide Mountain, and Mt. Rose. Below the trail are terraces built more than a half century ago in an effort to control flooding and slow the melting of snow.

The trail then climbs for a short distance before reaching a junction at about 0.5 mile from the junction of the dirt road, old TRT, and bike route at the Mt. Rose Wilderness boundary. Here an out-and-back trail climbs to the top of Mt. Houghton (see side trip "Mount Houghton").

From the junction with the Mt. Houghton Trail, the TRT starts heading downhill on a long traverse across open ridgeline. You pass scattered whitebark pines, aromatic pennyroyal, and ground lupine before reaching a switchback, which is just before a gully and a large black volcanic rock formation. Now the trail heads gently down to the west, with more open views all the way south to Freel Peak above Lake Tahoe's south shore. You reach an interesting jumble of volcanic boulders where a small spring feeds a charming garden of flowers, including rock fringe.

Past the spring, you roll in and out of little gullies, before the trail turns to the east, the grade eases, and the hemlocks start to appear. Look for a few flat potential tentsites before you hit a dirt

SIDE TRIP **Mount Houghton**

While Mt. Houghton is more of a high point on a ridge than a true mountain, the views and the interesting lichen-covered rocks on the way up are certainly worth the trip. After a moderate climb of about a half mile, you reach the summit where views of the Bronco Creek drainage and the whole of the Mt. Rose Wilderness unfold before you to the north. From here you can wander east along the pleasantly gentle ridgetop until you reach a steep drop into a cirque. Far below is the saddle of the Mt. Rose Trail and the trail to the Mt. Rose Summit. Once you have enjoyed the view, retrace your steps back to the TRT.

SIDE TRIP **Mount Rose**

Mt. Rose, the Tahoe area's third highest peak, is 2.6 miles and 1700 feet of climbing from the TRT and Mt. Rose Trail junction. If you are up for a good climb, it is worth it as the views along the way and at the top are extraordinary. Mt. Rose is unique in several ways and has a superb "garden" of alpine plants, including the woody fruited evening primrose, which is found almost exclusively on its slopes. This low-lying plant produces one or more large yellow blossoms on short stalks close to the ground. The flowers, which are pollinated by nocturnal moths and then die shortly afterward, smell like coconuts.

Mt. Rose also seems to have its own weather pattern. Often you can hike in shorts and a short-sleeve shirt until the last treeless 0.5 mile, where you encounter fierce winds and chilling temperatures. During a major winter blizzard, the top of Mt. Rose is truly frightening. The easiest way to the top of Mt. Rose is to start at the Mt. Rose and TRT Trailhead, which makes for a 10-mile round-trip with a little less than 2000 feet of climbing.

road and a junction. From here a right turn takes you a hundred yards to the dirt road and former TRT trail that comes down from Relay Peak. From there a left turn takes you past Snow Pond on the dirt road to the Mt. Rose Trailhead in about 3 miles.

A left turn from the new TRT junction takes you past a stream and wildflowers in 0.7 mile to a junction with the Mt. Rose Summit Trail. Straight ahead on the main TRT, you cross the faint road and head toward Galena Falls through forest. It starts out fairly level and then becomes a gentle descent through whitebark pines. There are several excellent level campsites above the trail. To your left you see meadows and Mt. Rose looming high above. At an open area with flat rocks, you can sit a spell and gaze up at the Relay Peak towers and see where you have been the last 3 miles. The trail soon reaches the top of Galena Falls, where flat rocks make an enticing spot to lie back, enjoy the views, and the sound of cascading water. The water for these falls springs out of the ground a few hundred yards upstream. While until now, this section of trail has been lightly used, expect crowds. The Mt. Rose Trailhead is one of the busiest in Nevada, and the bulk of the folks hike the easy 2.5 miles from the Mt. Rose Highway to the falls.

From here the trail switchbacks down through thick hemlock forest to the bottom of the falls and another trail junction. If there is a shortcoming with the Tahoe Rim Trail it is a lack of water, especially on the east side of the lake, so take a minute to relax by these glorious falls while deciding where to head next. For a special experience, come here in the autumn when cold temperatures create a border of ice on both sides of the falls.

If you turn left at the falls, you are now on the Mt. Rose Summit Trail, which quickly crosses Galena Creek and then skirts a meadow, before a gentle rise brings you across another creek and to a junction. Here a right turn takes you up to the top of Mt. Rose (see side trip "Mount Rose"). A left turn takes you over the creek you just crossed and then on a moderately steep ascent past a wonderful display of midsummer wildflowers. You reach the junction with the TRT that descends from Relay Peak in 0.7 mile. Going straight here would take you quickly to the Relay Peak dirt road and Snow Pond.

Back at the falls, the TRT goes straight ahead and circles above a large meadow. It then heads on a gently rising traverse below the slopes of beautiful, volcanic Tamarack Peak. The well-laid-out trail passes awesome views of Mt. Rose and Tamarack Lake. At about 2 miles from Galena Falls, a wide panorama of Lake Tahoe and Tahoe Meadows opens up before a gentle downhill traverse to

Rim to Reno Trail Network

Still under construction in 2011, the Rim to Reno Trail network is a major effort to connect Reno and the Tahoe Rim Trail via a network of trails. When it is completed in the next few years, hikers will be able to start at the Thomas Creek Trailhead, just off the Mt. Rose Highway on Timberline Drive, and hike to the saddle between Mt. Rose and Mt. Houghton, before descending to the Tahoe Rim Trail at Galena Falls.

As of fall 2011, more than 10 miles have been constructed from Thomas Creek, with perhaps another 10 to go. Also off of Timberline Drive, in the Mt. Rose Wilderness, is the 9-mile Jones Creek and Whites Creek Loop out of the Jones Creek Trailhead. This trail also connects to the Rim to Reno Trail via the Dry Pond Trail. In addition, a yet unnamed 7.5-mile loop, that includes a portion of the Rim to Reno Trail, has been built in the northwest section of the Mt. Rose Wilderness. While a primary goal of the trail building effort is to connect the Tahoe Rim Trail to the outskirts of Reno, this network of trails provides hikers access to the spectacular, but little-used Mt. Rose Wilderness. If you would like to help build this trail, contact the Tahoe Rim Trail Association for more information.

the Mt. Rose Summit Trailhead. This trailhead facility is located at the very top of the Mt. Rose Highway, across the street from the Mt. Rose Campground. It has pit toilets and parking. Thru-hikers can cross the highway to the campground, walk along the paved road for about a quarter mile and then hike an almost level 0.8 mile on the Tahoe Meadows Interpretative Trail to the Tahoe Meadows Trailhead.

Tahoe Meadows to Spooner Summit

(23.1 miles)

Difficulty This section is strenuous, mostly because of how long it is, but also because of the elevation gain. While the trail starts at 8740 feet and ends at about 7140 feet, there are two portions of the trail where you encounter climbs of more than 700 feet. In the opposite direction, the climb from Spooner Summit to just below Snow Valley Peak is about 1800 feet.

Best Seasons It is best to hike this section of the trail between mid-June and late October. The segment between Spooner Summit and Snow Valley Peak may be open as early as mid-May in years with light snowfall. However, the section between Twin Lakes and Snow Valley Peak may hold snow well into July.

Highlights There are spectacular vistas of Lake Tahoe along much of this section of trail. Some of these are the most stunning views to be found anywhere along the Tahoe Rim Trail. In particular, the Christopher's Loop (Herlan Peak) spur trail offers especially remarkable vistas. The trail provides views on both sides of this north-south oriented ridge, of Lake Tahoe to the west, and of the Great Basin to the east. While the thin decomposed granite soils along the trail limit wildflower growth, several locations have flowers in abundance. This is especially the case if you take a side trip down to Marlette Lake, where the wildflower display is one of the best to be found anywhere. If you are looking for yellow and orange aspen leaves, it is hard to beat the bounty of leaves at Snow Valley, Marlette Lake, and Spooner Lake.

Much of this section of trail can be covered on a mountain bike and, for the experienced rider, affords some of the best mountain biking at Lake Tahoe. This section of trail is home to the Tahoe Rim Trail 50-km, 50-mile, and 100-mile run that occurs in July.

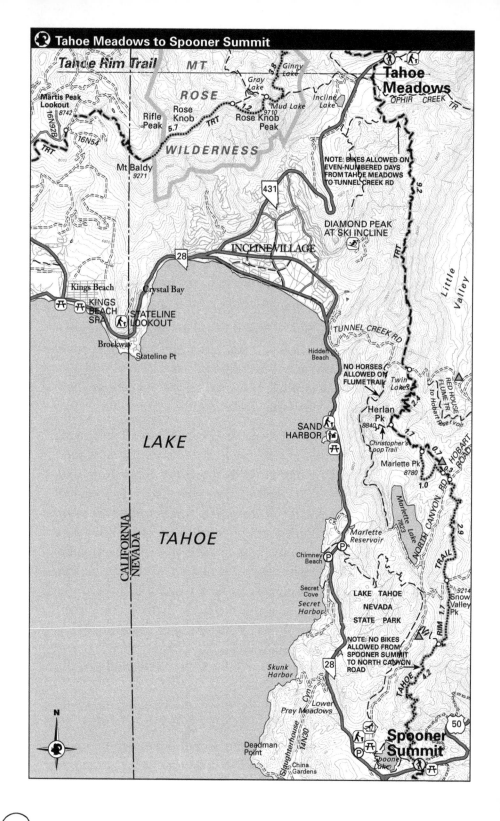

Tahoe Rim Trail

MT
ROSE
WILDERNESS

Ginny Lake
3.8
Gray Lake
Mud Lake
9710
Incline Lake

Tahoe Meadows
OPHIR CREEK TR

Martis Peak Lookout
8742
16N92B

Rose Knob
Rifle Peak
Rose Knob Peak
5.7
TRT

16N54

TRT
8000

Mt Baldy
9271

6800

6800

6000

NOTE: BIKES ALLOWED ON EVEN-NUMBERED DAYS FROM TAHOE MEADOWS TO TUNNEL CREEK RD

9.2

TRT

431

DIAMOND PEAK AT SKI INCLINE

INCLINE VILLAGE

28

Little Valley

Kings Beach
KINGS BEACH SRA

Crystal Bay
STATELINE LOOKOUT

Brockway

Stateline Pt

TUNNEL CREEK RD

Hidden Beach

NO HORSES ALLOWED ON FLUME TRAIL

Twin Lakes

2.4

RED HOUSE FLUME TR.
to Hobart Reservoir

LAKE

TAHOE

Herlan Pk
8840

to Hobart

1.7

SAND HARBOR

Christopher's Loop Trail

HOBART ROAD

0.7

Marlette Pk
8780

0.3

1.0

CALIFORNIA
NEVADA

Marlette Lake
7823

NORTH CANYON RD

2.9

Marlette Reservoir

Chimney Beach
P

P

LAKE TAHOE

NEVADA

STATE PARK

9214
Snow Valley Pk

Secret Cove

Secret Harbor

RIM

TRAIL

1.7

N

Skunk Harbor

28

NOTE: NO BIKES ALLOWED FROM SPOONER SUMMIT TO NORTH CANYON ROAD

TAHOE

4.2

Cpn

Lower Prey Meadows

Slaughterhouse
14N30

Deadman Point

China Gardens

Spooner Summit

Spooner Lake

P

50

As their slogan says, it truly is a glimpse of heaven and a taste of hell. For more information go to **www.tahoemtnmilers.org.**

Heads Up! There is very little water available on this section of trail. Bring some along for Fido. About 0.7 mile beyond the Tahoe Meadows Trailhead, you cross Ophir Creek, a beautiful little stream. At around mile 3 you pass two unreliable seasonal springs. At about 9.5 miles from the trailhead you reach the Twin Lakes. These two small, very shallow lakes may dry up by late in the summer; as they shrink, the water becomes less attractive and takes on a green hue. The hand-pump well at Marlette Campground, 13.8 miles from Tahoe Meadows, is the best source for water on this section. Another source for water is Spooner Lake, near Spooner Summit.

If you're thru-hiking, note that there are no trailside sources of water on the next 12 miles south of Spooner Summit. Obtain water at Spooner Lake unless you have made prior arrangements for water to be provided to you. While Spooner Lake's water itself looks marshy, you can also walk over to the Spooner Lake parking lot above the lake. Here you will find tap water and restrooms. You will see Marlette Lake from the trail. If you are thirsty or looking for a swim, it may be a worthwhile detour. From the intersection of the TRT and Hobart Road, it is 1.75 miles to the lake, mostly steep downhill. About 0.75 mile down, where two gullies converge, there is a usually reliable stream.

Most of the trail is exposed to the sun and wind so bring extra water, extra clothing, and lots of sunscreen. Camping is only allowed in two locations: One site, Marlette Peak Campground, is along the TRT near Marlette Peak, about 13 miles south of the Mt. Rose Trailhead; the second campsite is along North Canyon Road. At a minor saddle, just before you reach Snow Valley Peak, take a dirt road 1.2 miles steeply down to North Canyon Road. Turn left and go about 1 mile south down to North Canyon Campground, just east above the road. All you will see is an outhouse, with campsites behind it out of view from the road. Get

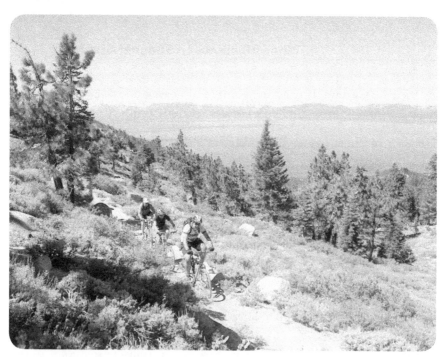

Mountain bikes between Tahoe Meadows and Tunnel Creek

water from the stream just to the west of the road. You can also continue on the TRT, past Snow Valley Peak an additional 1.7 miles, to a signed junction with a connector trail, which heads downhill 1.4 miles to the campground.

Tips for Mountain Bikers For the experienced mountain biker, this section of trail is perhaps the finest section on the entire Tahoe Rim Trail. It is best to ride from north to south. The Forest Service has ruled that mountain bikers should only use the northernmost 9.2 miles of this section of trail (from Mt. Rose Highway to Tunnel Creek Road) on even days of the month so that hikers may experience the trail without bikers on the odd days of the month. On an even weekend day in the middle of the summer, be prepared to see as many as 100 bikes.

After an initial fun ride across the meadow and then along the old Ophir Creek Trail, you turn right and climb to a saddle. Then it is a wonderful, sometimes challenging ride, mostly downhill, for the next 8 miles to Tunnel Creek Road. The trail is sandy and soft in some sections, but in most places it is firm and a real pleasure to ride. Some will feel challenged by portions of the trail; for most, the trouble is well rewarded.

At Tunnel Creek Road you can turn right and ride downhill 3 miles to Highway 28 where you can have a shuttle awaiting you. Or you can cross Tunnel Creek Road and head a short distance to Twin Lakes. The next few miles after Twin Lakes are a challenging steep uphill ride, but well worth the effort since they eventually lead to spectacular views of Marlette Lake and Lake Tahoe. When you reach Hobart Road, turn right. Bikes are *not* allowed on the rest of this section of the TRT. Hobart Road takes you down to Marlette Lake, where you follow North Canyon Road out to the parking lot at Lake Tahoe Nevada State Park, where fees are required for parking or for riding through the park.

Getting There, Highway 431 (Mt. Rose Highway) to Spooner Summit The trailhead is 7.3 miles north on Highway 431 (toward Reno) from the junction of Highways 28 and 431 in Incline Village. You will drive past Tahoe Meadows on your right to a parking area and restroom facility on your right. The trail starts from the western edge of the lower parking lot. From Reno, this trailhead is found about 0.75 mile after the highway tops the Mt. Rose Summit.

Getting There, Spooner Summit to Highway 431 (Mt. Rose Highway) From Tahoe City you travel 27 miles east on Highway 28 to reach the junction with Highway 50. Turn left on Highway 50, and drive 0.7 mile to the trailhead on the north (left) side of the road (approximately 14 miles northeast of South Lake Tahoe on Highway 50). There is a small paved parking area on the north side of the highway, situated across from a larger paved parking lot, which provides access to the southbound TRT. It is important to realize that Spooner Summit is not the same as Spooner Lake. Spooner Lake is about 0.5 mile west of the junction of Highways 50 and 28 on Highway 28. Entrance to the popular Spooner Lake area (with access to the Flume Trail) requires a fee; to reach it drive 0.6 mile northwest from the junction.

Trail Description

From Highway 431, known locally as the Mt. Rose Highway, the southbound TRT runs parallel to the highway and descends past several streamlets and then crosses through the middle of Tahoe Meadows, a large subalpine area that can be muddy in June or a wonderful wildflower tromp in July. Stay on the trail to avoid damaging the fragile meadow ecosystem. Near the south edge of the meadow, cross Ophir Creek, a charming year-round stream that is bordered by elephant heads, lupines, and other wildflowers. Except for the fact that you just left the trailhead 0.75 mile ago it would be the best source for water on this section of trail. After crossing Ophir Creek on the wide bridge, the trail heads into a forest of lodgepole and whitebark pines, and meets the Ophir Creek Trail, where you turn left (south). For the next 0.2 mile, you are walking past lodgepole pines on a smooth, wide trail. Soon to the left you see Tahoe Meadows and the radio towers atop Slide Mountain, before the trail meets a junction 1 mile from the trailhead. For information on the network of trails heading out from the Ophir Creek Bridge refer to the side trip "Tahoe Meadows."

> ### SIDE TRIP Tahoe Meadows
>
> Three interconnected loop trails provide access to the beauty of Tahoe Meadows. They are popular easy hikes for families and people with dogs. The longest is 3 miles, with about half in the trees using the TRT and Ophir Creek Trails, and the other half on the edge of the meadow where you can hear and see the creek. A section of the trail near the TRT bridge is on boardwalk, which protects the fragile meadow from damage while allowing walkers to get very close to the narrow, but deep creek. A connector trail leads along the east side of the creek from the TRT directly to Highway 431, providing a shorter route to the meadow trails. There is a map of the different routes adjacent to the bridge.

Straight ahead is the Ophir Creek Trail. It starts out level in the lodgepole forest and then heads downhill, sometimes steeply, past prolific groves of aspen trees and western white pines to the backside of Slide Mountain.

In 3 miles on the Ophir Creek Trail you reach what remains of Upper Price Lake, which was significantly reduced in size by

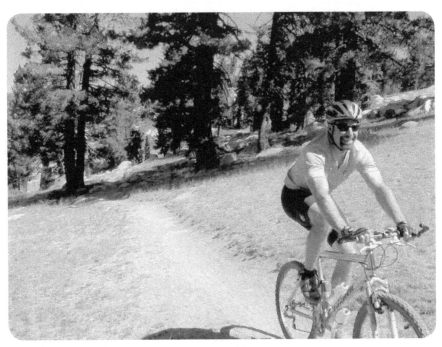

Happy biker near Tahoe Meadows

a landslide in 1983. This is a great trail for fall colors and to see how Slide Mountain got its name. It also seems to be a very popular area for hang gliders. One beautiful fall day I sat mesmerized by the antics of eight gliders riding the thermals above Slide Mountain. Eventually you reach Davis Creek County Park in 7 miles, although most will find the venture to Upper Price Lake and back a better way to spend their time.

The TRT turns right and starts a gentle climb south up the sandy surface past more scattered lodgepole pines and occasional western white pines and whitebark pines. Exposed to high winds and heavy snows on this north-facing slope, the trees are smaller than those you will see later on the south-facing side of the ridge. To the north you can see the rose-colored top of Mt. Rose.

At 1.7 miles from the trailhead you reach a saddle, about 250 feet above the Ophir Creek Trail. Here you get your first views of Lake Tahoe through the vegetation. The views just keep getting better and better as the miles go by. Now your pathway is along a long north-south oriented ridge for the next 7.5 miles, going in and out of the tops of east-west oriented gullies. Along the route

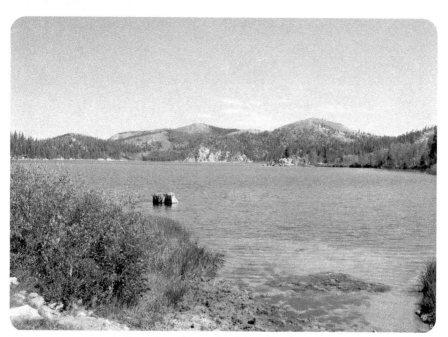
Looking toward Marlette Peak from Marlette Lake

you will experience numerous gentle ups and downs, and from the saddle have an overall drop in altitude of about 900 feet to Tunnel Creek Road.

The first mile past the saddle is a gentle, sandy contour along the western slope of the ridge. You pass scattered white granite boulders, appearing as if they were tossed there haphazardly by a giant playing with rocks. Lodgepole pines are now fewer and larger, and there are some impressively large western white pines with their long narrow cones hanging from the top. Some may mistake the western white pines for sugar pines, but the sugar pine cones are quite a bit larger, and sugar pines are usually found at lower elevations. At 2.5 miles from the trailhead you cross the head of a gully; here the trail changes from its eastern direction to a southern direction. You see a wide view of the lake, looking toward Emerald Bay and Mt. Tallac. Several large, flat granite boulders just below the trail make this a great spot to sit and enjoy the views.

Next you ascend gently and enjoy more views of the lake looking toward the Nevada and California border, which lies on a large peninsula jutting straight south into the lake. Soon, about

3 miles from the trailhead, you reach two spring-fed streamlets and colorful lush vegetation, which provide a cool break from the dry, sandy terrain that surrounds the area. The trail next winds up and down past a few hemlock trees before reaching another saddle 3.6 miles from the trailhead with views of Mt. Rose to the north. You then begin a short moderately steep descent over a number of evenly spaced granite steps (a joy for the experienced mountain biker), followed by a short climb to another viewpoint.

Every half mile you walk provides an even wider and more beautiful view of the lake. On a clear windy day, the wind ripples shimmer in the sun as the lake turns a deep blue. At a little more than 4 miles from the trailhead, your trail now crosses to the east-facing side of the ridge, passing a flat opening with stumps from ancient logging. Here you get your first glimpse of Washoe Lake and the Great Basin to the east. A gentle descent leads to a wider opening with a view of all of Washoe Lake.

At 4.6 miles from your Tahoe Meadows Trailhead you go southwest, gently uphill, followed by a moderate descent, back to the west-facing slope. Here where the trail takes a sharp left turn, you find another viewpoint just off the trail to your right. Again, several flat boulders provide a resting spot to appreciate the views. Southwest across Lake Tahoe you see Twin Peaks (8878 feet), prominent above the northwest shore, and to the southwest, Emerald Bay and behind it, Maggies Peaks (8699 feet and 8499 feet). Incline Village lies directly below you to the west.

Past this viewpoint you travel into a thicker forest of red firs and scattered western white pines as you cross to the east-facing side of the ridge once again. Soon, you reach a trail hanging on the edge of the steep bank and pass just to the east of the top of a Diamond Peak Ski Area lift, before reaching a saddle at 5.7 miles from the trailhead. Here you find wide open, east-facing views toward Carson City and Washoe Lake. The trail next bends to the west and Lake Tahoe so dominates your senses that it appears as if you could walk right into it. Jeffrey pines now predominate, as you head down a short, steep rock staircase (many bikers will want to get off their bikes, others will wish they had halfway down). The long ridge that includes Mt. Baldy, Rose Knob Peak, and Relay Peak can be seen to your north. Below you to the west are the ski runs and condominium developments of Diamond Peak Ski Area, the town of Incline Village, and the Incline area golf courses.

About 1 mile past the Diamond Peak ski lift, the trail climbs through granite boulders to the eastern slope again. Here you pass from the land of Jeffrey pines to the land of red firs and meander up and down gently through the forest before reaching another viewpoint opening through the trees to the east. About 7 miles from your trailhead, you start a moderate descent on a long switchback. If you are hiking, you will enjoy views to the east of Little Valley and Washoe Lake. If you are on a bike, you will be hanging on, trying not to lose your balance on the deep, soft sand. From the bottom of the descent, you pass ground-hugging pinemat manzanita and chinquapin, briefly head through a fir forest, and then end up back out on a mostly treeless west-facing slope, about 8 miles into your hike.

> ### SIDE TRIP **Flume Trail**
>
> A left turn here soon takes you downhill steeply on the Red House Flume Trail, a popular bike loop in combination with the Flume Trail. A right turn takes you downhill steeply for 0.5 mile to a junction with the Flume Trail. From this junction, a left turn will take you on the Flume Trail (although it is recommended that you ride the Flume Trail the opposite direction, starting from Spooner Lake), a right turn goes down Tunnel Creek Road steeply for 2.6 miles to Highway 28.

The final stage of your journey to Tunnel Creek Road is a gentle up and down through a moderately dense forest of red and white firs on a trail cut out of the side of the ridge. Views of the lake are mostly filtered, with one last dramatic viewpoint to the west toward the beaches of Incline Village, Twin Peaks, Dollar Point, and the Lake Forest "island" (a peninsula during low water periods, an island during high-water periods). Highway 267 can be seen climbing over the top of Brockway Summit.

Marlette Lake and Lake Tahoe from Snow Valley Peak

At Tunnel Creek Road, 9.2 miles from your trailhead, you meet a junction with the Red House Flume Trail. Now you are in an area that is very busy with mountain bikers much of the year. If you are hiking, keep your eyes open for riders; if you are riding, watch out for hikers (see side trip "Flume Trail").

To continue on the Tahoe Rim Trail, go straight through level terrain about 0.3 mile to the lower of the two Twin Lakes. These lakes have been the location of several backcountry camps sponsored by mountain biking groups and the Tahoe Rim Trail Association who use the camps as they work to maintain and improve the trail. These shallow grass-lined lakes may dry up by midsummer after most winters. If you're desperate for water, the higher of the Twin Lakes, not visible from the trail, dries up later than the lower lake.

From the east shore of Lower Twin Lake, you face a 1.5-mile long, 750-foot climb, usually moderate, but sometimes steep, through a mixed forest of pine and fir trees. With its soft sand surface, this trail feels steeper on a bike. There are occasional views of Mt. Rose back to the north and Lake Tahoe to the west. After a series of switchbacks, you almost reach the top of Peak 8706.

SIDE TRIP **Christopher's Loop Trail**

This 1.2-mile loop trail is well worth the climb. The trail switch-backs steeply up to the top of a sandy ridge. Now you are at the top, but the best viewpoint is still a bit of a walk west toward the lake. Your trail goes across an open pla-teau and in a fairly short distance reaches Christopher's Loop. Go left since the right side doesn't receive much use and is less maintained.

Once you are there, you are stand-ing on a granite cliff looking down on Sand Harbor while the entire lake unfolds before you. It is the best view of Lake Tahoe I have seen anywhere. The first time you see it, your jaw will drop in amazement. The view to the south of Marlette Lake and Snow Valley Peak is also spectacular. This is a great spot to stop for lunch, although since it is about 12 miles from the trailhead, you must get a very early start or bike instead of hike to get here by lunchtime. Backpackers hiking the trail counterclockwise can spend the night at Marlette Campground and then be at the viewpoint for an excellent photo opportunity within an hour of leaving camp in the morning.

Traverse west below it, then go south downhill into a level open area, before traversing briefly west and climbing again. This climb is shorter, a mere 0.25 mile, and just before leveling off, you reach a junction at about 2.4 miles from the trail intersection with Tunnel Creek Road. This is the Christopher's Loop spur view trail on Herlan Peak. If you are on your bike, leave it here as bikes are *not* allowed on this viewpoint loop (see side trip "Christopher's Loop Trail").

You are now about halfway through the TRT's Section 3. Heading southeast on the TRT you find that the route has leveled off before it enters an area that is thick with hemlock trees, which can hold the snow until early summer. A short distance farther, you pass through a flat area of scattered pine trees before reach-ing a wide open, treeless ridgetop. Here, about 0.75 mile beyond Christopher's Loop, walk about 100 yards south on a use trail, which ends with inspiring views of most of Marlette Lake in the foreground and Lake Tahoe in the background. Nearby, Marlette Peak and Snow Valley Peak are visible to the south.

The trail now heads east and down to the eastern slope of the ridge to an area thick with some especially large lupine and paint-brush plants. Stop and gaze east for another view over the flowers to the Great Basin. When you continue, you descend along the

Sand Harbor from Christopher's Loop

east-facing slope past grassy areas with more wildflowers and forested areas of red fir and hemlock. This is a wonderfully enjoyable rolling stretch on a mountain bike. You meet a trail junction at 1.7 miles from the Christopher's Loop junction.

From here you have two alternative TRT routes to choose from. The trail to the right is for hikers only; in 1 mile it traverses the west and south slopes of Marlette Peak, providing panoramic full views of Marlette Lake, Snow Valley Peak, and Lake Tahoe. A left turn at the junction keeps you on the Tahoe Rim Trail, which continues to be multiple use here. You head through more rolling forested terrain and in 0.5 mile, meet the simple Marlette Peak campground with a pit toilet, food storage lockers, a few picnic tables, and water via a well. Just 0.2 mile farther the TRT meets the trail that circled Marlette Peak, and the trails are rejoined as one. So which route should you take? If you are riding your bike, please stick to the east section. If you are a hiker and would enjoy more sensational views, take the slightly longer (by 0.3 mile) Marlette Peak Trail.

From where your trails meet, you head 0.3 mile mostly downhill through open sandy terrain to a junction with Hobart Road.

SIDE TRIP **Marlette Lake**

If you need water or would enjoy a swim in a wonderful lake or if you are on a mountain bike, leave the Tahoe Rim Trail, turn right on Hobart Road, and head 2.1 miles down to a junction by the southeast shore of Marlette Lake, named after Seneca Hope Marlette, the first surveyor general of California and one of Tahoe's first mapmakers. Mountain bikes are *not* allowed on the remaining portion of this section of the TRT, so you must turn right if you are biking. Hobart Road is level for about 0.5 mile and then heads downhill steeply over some very soft decomposed granite to a flatter section of great riding past springtime wildflowers and aspen trees to the junction next to Marlette Lake. In the spring or early summer the east shore of Marlette Lake has one of the most prolific exhibits of wildflowers anywhere. More than 50 different species of flowers, including lupine, paintbrush, monkshood, horsemint, columbine, tiger lily, and elephant heads, are reported to be in this area.

From the junction, a short road descends to the southeast shore of Marlette Lake, where you can stop to swim, and then continue south on the main road on your left, which heads 0.7 mile moderately steeply up to the top of the saddle. From the saddle, follow North Canyon Road 3.9 miles on hard-packed sand down to the Spooner Lake parking lot. On a bike this is a fun downhill, but watch out for hikers and obey the speed limits—yes, speed limits (5 miles per hour on turns or when passing someone and 20 miles per hour anywhere else). If you are walking, bound for Spooner Lake via North Canyon and wish to avoid the bikers, take the new Marlette Lake Trail, where bikes are *not* allowed. It starts on the south end of the lake, near the main creek that drains into the lake, and heads 4.5 miles to the Spooner Lake parking lot. Along the trail you enjoy beautiful views of Snow Valley and Snow Valley Peak, lots of aspens, several streams, and the remnants of a logger's cabin. Next to the beginning of the Marlette Trail is a fish spawning station. To see the fish in action, visit this spot in June or early July.

At this junction if you would like to head to Marlette Lake, see side trip "Marlette Lake."

At the Hobart Road junction, which is about 14.3 miles from the Tahoe Meadows Trailhead and about 8.8 miles from the Spooner Summit Trailhead, the TRT crosses the road and begins the 2.9-mile, 700-foot climb to the saddle below Snow Valley Peak. Bikes are *not* allowed between Hobart Road and Spooner Summit on the Tahoe Rim Trail. Head initially east into the trees and soon begin a moderate ascent south. After about 0.7 mile, the TRT reaches a jeep road and follows it about 140 yards west before turning south again. If you are low on water, take this road

Marlette Lake and Lake Tahoe

0.2 mile southwest down a gully to where the road starts to climb northwest. Continue about 200 yards down the gully to a spring.

Beyond the jeep road your ascent gets steep as you journey through a forest of red firs and western white pines. You see occasional glimpses of Snow Valley Peak to the south and of Marlette Lake to your west. As you near the top of the ridge and Snow Valley Peak, there are fewer trees (a few windblown whitebark pines) and the views are more spectacular. You pass through expansive fields of lupine and sagebrush bordered by piles of granite rock boulders. To the north, you can see downtown Reno and its surrounding desert as well as Mt. Rose.

Just before reaching the saddle below Snow Valley Peak, the trail crosses to the west-facing side of the ridge, providing unobstructed views of Marlette Lake and Lake Tahoe. This viewpoint makes for a wonderful spot for lunch or rest before beginning the long descent to Spooner Summit. At a shallow notch by the northwest base of Snow Valley Peak, the TRT crosses a dirt road coming up from North Canyon below, the large valley and meadow area to the southwest (see side trip "Spooner Lake," next page).

From the junction of the TRT and this dirt road, you can also climb in 0.3 mile to the top of Snow Valley Peak, which at 9214 feet is the highest peak on the eastern slope of the Tahoe Basin. To get there follow the road east as it climbs up the mountain. The walk to the top of Snow Valley Peak requires an additional 270 feet of climbing for a view that to my mind is not as good as the one of Marlette Lake and Lake Tahoe you just passed, but peak baggers will have bagged a peak.

SIDE TRIP Spooner Lake

To go to Spooner Lake, turn right and in 1.2 miles of steep downhill you will reach a spring and then immediately North Canyon Road, where you turn left. From here, an additional 3.8 miles of a moderate, then gentle, downhill path takes you to Spooner Lake at the Lake Tahoe Nevada State Park parking area. Remember, that is Spooner Lake, not the Spooner *Summit* Trailhead parking lot for the Tahoe Rim Trail.

When you arrive at North Canyon Road after coming down from Snow Valley Peak, you could also take the Marlette Lake Trail to Spooner Lake or Marlette Lake. Cross the road and hike about 50 yards west to the Marlette Lake Trail. To go to Marlette Lake, turn right and go downhill about 0.5 mile to the lake. To go to Spooner Lake, turn left and go about 3 miles moderately steeply downhill to a junction with North Canyon Road. Cross the road and follow the pathway another 0.5 mile to the Spooner Lake parking lot and nearby lake.

If you stay on the Rim Trail heading south, you will hike 5.9 miles from the junction with the dirt road to the trailhead at Spooner Summit. The first mile is a rambling gentle downhill across an exposed ridge with sagebrush, tobacco brush, lots of granite boulders, and a few stunted whitebark pines. You get expansive views of Lake Tahoe, as well as views of the North Canyon Road and a vast forest of aspen trees. The view is especially spectacular in the fall with a sea of yellow aspen leaves. Enjoy the open view because soon you will be in a dense forest. If you have a pair of binoculars, you can count the numerous bikers grunting their way up the steep North Canyon route toward Marlette Lake, as well as those on the ever popular Flume Trail.

In this area, several very charming log cabins close to the Tahoe Rim Trail are available for rental year-round, as well as a shuttle service for mountain bikers and hikers using the Flume Trail or the Tahoe Rim Trail. For more information about renting cabins contact Nevada State Parks at (775) 831-0494. For infor-

Looking south from Christopher's Loop

mation about shuttle services, contact Flume Trail Bikes at (775) 749-5349 or visit **www.theflumetrail.com**. They operate shuttle services from Tunnel Creek Station, at the end of the Flume Trail in Incline, where they provide food and rental bikes.

After an abundance of Lake Tahoe views, the trail ventures to the east-facing side of the ridge for views of Eagle Valley, with its sprawling Carson City. Then you head into a thick forest of red fir and Jeffrey pine as the trail continues down the ridge. Along this ridgeline section, as you may have seen earlier on the trail, are old weathered stumps cut as high as five to six feet off the ground. These trees were cut in the 1870s to provide wood for the Marlette Flume below Marlette Lake, from where the wood traveled by water to Carson City, and eventually Virginia City, to support the silver mines. The dry climate of the east shore has kept the stumps from decomposing over all these years. At 1.7 miles from the junction with the trail to the top of Snow Valley Peak, you meet a junction on a minor saddle. From here, a trail descends northwest, losing more than 700 feet in elevation as it switchbacks in 1.4 miles to primitive North Canyon Campground and adjacent North Canyon Road. Near this campground, there

Christopher's Loop

is water at a small creek that flows through a grove of aspens just west of the road.

On the TRT, with a little more than 4 miles to go, your trail now winds gently downhill along a heavily forested ridgeline of pine and fir trees. The trail is soft dirt and an easy walk (although if you are doing this whole route in one day, it may not seem easy at this point). Occasional filtered views open up, but this is primarily a walk through a shady forest. At 1.4 miles south of the campground trail junction, a vista trail leads off to the right. After a 100-yard jaunt up this spur trail, you will find views of Lake Tahoe and the mountains above the lake's west shore. If you started hiking from the Spooner Summit Trailhead, this vista point is 2.8 miles from the trailhead and 1000 feet above it.

Your gentle-to-moderate walk winds through the forest pathway for another 2.25 miles before ending with a short steep descent to a dirt road. On it the TRT turns left, and you walk 0.5 mile, passing a large grove of aspen trees with filtered views of Spooner Lake to the end of the section.

Alternative Routes

Do you like beautiful views but do not feel ready for a 23-mile jaunt? These alternative routes are shorter but still reach some great viewpoints.

- Start at the Tahoe Meadows Trailhead, and hike as far as you want and then turn around. You will find an abundance of great viewpoints and numerous lunch spots on the flat granite rocks. This relatively easy trip is an excellent route for families hiking with children.

- Start at Tahoe Meadows, and hike 9.2 miles south to where the TRT runs into Tunnel Creek Road. Turn right (west) and walk or ride steeply downhill for 3.1 miles to Highway 28. Be careful going downhill since the sand can be quite deep, especially later in the summer and fall. If you time it correctly, the fall colors in Tunnel Creek Canyon can be spectacular. Shuttle service may be available through Flume Trail Bikes, (775) 749-5349.

- Start at the Spooner North Trailhead, and hike 5.9 miles to the saddle below Snow Valley Peak where you meet a dirt road. Turn left and follow this road 1.2 miles to where it intersects the North Canyon Road. Turn left again and walk 3.8 miles to the Spooner Lake parking lot. You can then walk around Spooner Lake and find a trail to the Spooner Summit parking area.

Spooner Summit to Kingsbury Grade

(18.5 miles)

Difficulty Moderately difficult. There is a steady climb of about 1600 feet in the first 5 miles and a wonderful almost level mile in the middle, filled with views. Then the trail is mostly downhill. The starting elevation is 7150 feet, and the ending elevation is 7780 feet, with the high point just a little below the top of South Camp Peak (8866 feet).

Best Seasons Early June to late October. The east shore gets less snow, and it melts faster here than the west shore, so this is a good choice for early season hiking. There are several heavily forested north-facing sections that may retain snow until late June, but in most areas the snow melts by late May.

Highlights The biggest highlight of this section is the spectacular view of most of Lake Tahoe and the west shore from South Camp Peak. This unobstructed view looks directly up the entrance of Emerald Bay to the mountains of Desolation Wilderness. At South Camp Peak you will find lots of rocks to sit on and even a wood bench that some kind trail builder provided. This could be the perfect TRT lunch spot. Making South Camp Peak your turnaround point for an out-and-back hike or ride makes good sense whether you are starting from the Spooner Summit Trailhead or from Kingsbury Grade. The new section of the TRT near Kingsbury Grade completed in 2012 allows the thru-hiker to avoid walking several miles on paved residential streets and provides miles of interesting new trail that has immediately become popular.

Heads Up! Water is not available between Spooner Summit and the Kingsbury North Trailhead. Several streams provide water between Kingsbury North and Kingsbury South. Be sure to bring

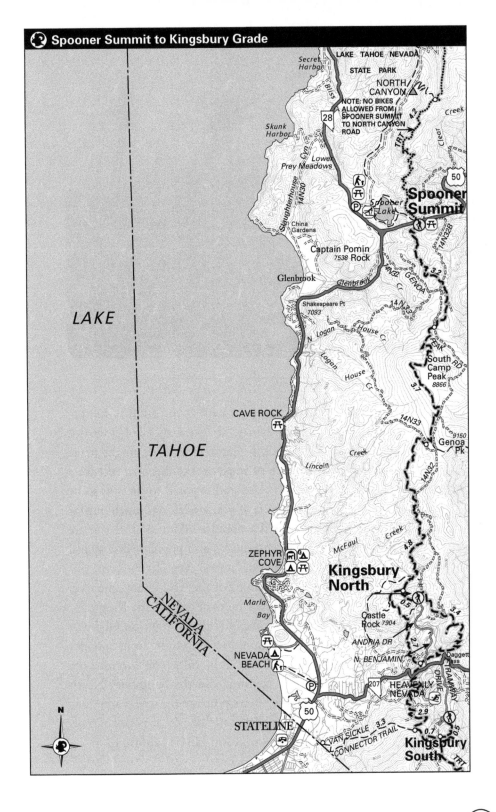

LAKE TAHOE NEVADA

STATE PARK

Secret Harbor

NORTH CANYON

NOTE: NO BIKES ALLOWED FROM SPOONER SUMMIT TO NORTH CANYON ROAD

28

4.2

Creek

Skunk Harbor

Clear Creek

TRT

Lower Prey Meadows

14N30

Slaughterhouse Cyn

Spooner Lake

P

50

Spooner Summit

14N32B

China Gardens

Captain Pomin 7538 Rock

3.2

GENOA

ANGL CR

Glenbrook

Glenbrook

14N33

Shakespeare Pt 7093

N Logan

House Cr

PEAK

South Camp Peak 8866

Logan

House Cr

3.7

CAVE ROCK

14N33

9150

Genoa Pk

Creek

Lincoln

14N32

McFaul

Creek

4.8

ZEPHYR COVE

Kingsbury North

Marla Bay

0.5

3.4

Castle Rock 7904

ANDRIA DR

2.1

NEVADA CALIFORNIA

N. BENJAMIN

Daggett Pass

NEVADA BEACH

P

207

TRAMWAY DRIVE

HEAVENLY NEVADA

2.9

N

50

STATELINE

VAN SICKLE 3.3 CONNECTOR TRAIL

0.7

0.5

Kingsbury South

TRT

LAKE

TAHOE

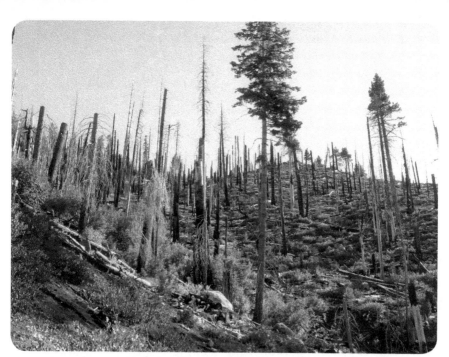

Van Sickle Trail

plenty of water for yourself and your pets. If you are thru-hiking, be sure to fill your water containers at Spooner Lake before you reach the trailhead. While South Camp Peak itself might make a good camping spot, the lack of water makes this hike best for a day trip. Much of the trail is open and exposed to the sun so be sure to bring plenty of sunscreen. If you are hiking, watch out for mountain bikers because this is a popular biking trail. If you are biking, watch out for hikers because it's also popular with hikers. Both groups should *watch* out for horses. *Note:* In the past, this was the shortest of the eight sections of the TRT—not anymore. The addition of more than 12 new miles of trails in the Kingsbury Grade area and the lack of an official trailhead right on Highway 207 makes the official TRT section now 18.5 miles from Spooner Summit to Kingsbury Grade South. It is still possible to hike the 12.2 miles between Spooner Summit and the Kingsbury North Trailhead. If you have hiked this section before the recent additions to the trail, read this new description carefully; the network of trails in the Kingsbury area is complicated and can be confusing.

Tips for Mountain Bikers Mountain bikes are allowed on this entire section. This ride can be completed from either direction, with the impressive views of South Camp Peak in the middle making a good location for a break. The section from Spooner to South Camp Peak is a great ride. It is an easy-to-moderate climb most of the way on smooth and sandy trails. If you get to the top and turn around, the downhill is a thrill—fun but not too difficult. The section from South Camp Peak to Kingsbury is more technical because of rocky steps and challenging terrain.

Getting There, Spooner Summit to Kingsbury From the "Y" in Tahoe City, drive 27 miles east on Highway 28 past Incline Village to the top of Spooner Summit, where Highway 28 meets Highway 50. Turn left on Highway 50, and drive 0.7 mile to the trailhead parking lot on the right, which has room for 20 cars. The Spooner-to-Kingsbury Trailhead has a pit toilet and several picnic tables in a nice setting under a grove of aspen trees. The trailhead is about 14 miles northeast of South Lake Tahoe on Highway 50. Directly across Highway 50 is the Spooner-to-Highway 431 Trailhead.

Getting There, Kingsbury North to Spooner Summit From Highway 50 at Stateline, Nevada, drive 2.9 miles up (east) Highway 207 (Kingsbury Grade), and turn left on North Benjamin Drive. (This is 0.3 mile before the top of Daggett Pass.) North Benjamin becomes Andria Drive, and you go a total of 1.9 miles from the highway to the end of the pavement and a trailhead with the Tahoe Rim Trail sign on your left.

Getting There, Kingsbury South to Spooner Summit Follow directions as above, but continue past North Benjamin and turn right on Tramway when you reach the top of Kingsbury Grade. Follow Tramway, 1.5 miles to the Kingsbury South Trailhead at the Stagecoach parking lot.

Trail Description

From Spooner Summit, the mostly sandy trail climbs moderately up a somewhat open slope where manzanita, chinquapin, tobacco brush, and sagebrush grow. In a fairly short time, the grade eases, and you begin a steady, but less steep, climb through open forest, meadows, and thicker stands of Jeffrey pines and red firs. Here, the trail is smooth, hard-packed sand, which is wonderful for mountain bikers. This open forest is a popular area for both deer and bear, and mountain lions have also been spotted in the area. During the drought of the early 1990s, a high percentage of trees in the area died because they lacked the necessary moisture to fight off invading bark beetles. In the late 1990s the area was logged heavily to remove the dead trees. The result has been a more open forest and some new dramatic views of the surrounding mountains.

Along the way south toward South Camp Peak, you intermittently glimpse Lake Tahoe and Desolation Wilderness to the west, and Snow Valley Peak to the north. Mules ears, paintbrush, lupine, and several aspen groves grow along the trail. After about 550 feet of ascent and 1.5 miles, you reach a little knoll with a short spur trail to the top, providing views into the Carson Valley and to the north toward Snow Valley Peak (9214 feet) and Mt. Rose (10,776 feet), two mountains of the Carson Range. While enjoying the view, contemplate the Carson Range, which is the transition zone between two very different environments.

To the west, along the slopes above the western edge of Lake Tahoe, is the heart of the Sierra Nevada, where every winter copious amounts of snow fall. That area is lush with a thick forest, green meadows, and countless lakes. The snow lasts well into summer. Where you stand in the Carson Range, on the other hand, receives about half as much snow as the western slope does. The trees are more scattered and lakes are rare. The drier area that you see to the east is the edge of the basin and range high desert zone, which dominates most of Nevada and Utah. This area

Grubb viewpoint from Kingsbury Grade

receives considerably less annual precipitation than the Carson Range does. While many factors determine what the natural surroundings look like, in the western United States the biggest determining factor is how much precipitation an area receives.

About 0.6 mile past the spur trail, your route turns from south to east, and after a nearly level 0.4-mile traverse, it crosses a minor road about 250 yards north of where it ends at Genoa Peak Road, a major forest service road. A large aspen grove grows alongside it, but you won't find any flowing water. You've climbed only about 100 feet in the last mile, but now you turn southward and climb gently 0.4 mile to an abandoned road that would take you southeast in 0.25 mile to a pond that usually has water into June. After a second 0.4-mile climb, you reach a second short spur trail, which takes you to less spectacular views. Now you descend 0.3 mile west to a crossing of the major Genoa Peak Road, about 3.5 miles from the trailhead, adjacent to a large open staging area for logging operations.

The trail then becomes increasingly steeper as you begin an unrelenting 800-foot climb to the crest of South Camp Peak through heavily forested terrain. You may see signs of logging,

Genoa Peak from South Camp Peak

including numerous blackened stumps. The trees were cut down and the brush and debris from them was burned. Just before reaching the northwest edge of South Camp Peak, the trail passes through a thickly forested north-facing section where you may see snow in early summer.

South Camp Peak is a large, nearly level, open area with great picnic sites. You walk along the broad summit's west rim, and its low-lying shrubs do not obstruct the spectacular views, which you have for 1 mile. The summit is so broad and level in fact that *peak* is a misnomer. The highest rock outcropping is about 0.75 mile along your rim traverse, and looking southeast from it, you see Genoa Peak, the nearby pointy peak with a radio tower on top. Scanning clockwise, next you see Heavenly Ski Resort and beyond it to the south, brown, rounded Freel Peak; Stateline and its casinos, as well as the rest of the South Lake Tahoe area; evidence of the 2007 Angora Fire; Fallen Leaf Lake; Desolation Wilderness, including the pointy spire of Pyramid Peak; Mt. Tallac, which seems to rise up right from the lake; Emerald Bay and evidence of the landslide that occurred in 1955, just after the construction of Highway 89 along the bay. Next comes Stony Ridge, with Jacks

Peak and nipple-topped Rubicon Peak, and then to the west the deep westshore canyons: Blackwood and Ward (with Twin Peaks on the ridge between the two canyons). Increasingly northwest you see Alpine Meadows, Squaw Valley, and to their north, Castle Peak above Donner Summit. While the views are spectacular, sometimes the winds are ferocious as you gaze from this exposed lookout straight into prevailing westerly winds. From this angle you can see right into Emerald Bay and you may get the mistaken impression that Lake Tahoe is 100 miles long and 5 miles wide.

Unless you take a steep side trip up to Genoa Peak, South Camp Peak, at around 8800 feet, is the highest point along this section of trail. If you would like to hike an out-and-back on this section of the TRT, turn around here. It makes for a wonderful 10- to 12-mile round-trip (the mileage depends on where you turn around). If you complete the entire point-to-point route from Spooner Summit to Kingsbury Grade, you will probably drag yourself away from the views and start heading gently downhill and away from the sometimes stiff winds in the direction of Genoa Peak. In 0.5 mile you reach a saddle with a dirt road that climbs southeast to Genoa Peak (see side trip "Genoa Peak").

> **SIDE TRIP Genoa Peak**
>
> In 0.8 mile of steep climbing you will be at the top of Genoa Peak (9150 feet). The views of Lake Tahoe from the top of Genoa Peak are similar to those from South Camp Peak, but you get the added bonus of views of Carson Valley to the east. On the negative side, you will be standing next to a radio tower. The area around Genoa Peak is popular with glider planes. Once, I saw one fly by so close to the peak that the pilot and I could wave at each other.

On the TRT, from the junction with the Genoa Peak jeep road, you begin a 5-mile long and usually gentle descent toward the North Kingsbury Grade Trailhead. The forest here is composed primarily of small young Jeffrey pines, red firs, and western white pines, and you may continue to see the blackened stumps left behind by past logging. Pinemat manzanita, a luscious green ground cover, is especially prolific in this section and adds a nice green feel to the hike. About 0.7 mile past the road that led up to Genoa Peak, you cross a small dirt road on the floor of a gully, and here the trail turns northwest and then south as it rounds a peak. Just before passing this small dirt road, you meet a junction with the Sierra Canyon Trail (see side trip "Sierra Canyon Trail").

You traverse the mountainside on a trail that has become more challenging and technical for mountain bikers. Your path is now bordered by granite boulders, and you have many rock steps to climb over. The forest has become thicker, and so you get only occasional glimpses of the lake. One of these views, however, is a dramatic look at Emerald Bay and Mt. Tallac, which feels much closer to this section of trail. As you continue on a narrower, rocky trail, you see Heavenly Ski Resort and its accompanying development. The stark view of high-rise condominiums detracts from the feeling that you are away from it all.

The trail continues to roll up and down along short stretches until you meet a junction. Here a left turn takes you on the Kingsbury North Access Trail east 0.5 mile to the Kingsbury North Trailhead on Andria Drive. The main TRT heads straight ahead on a trail completed in 2011. After a short gentle climb, the trail winds through white firs and Jeffrey pines in a gentle descent. Just 0.4 mile past the Access Trail, the TRT meets the Kingsbury Stinger Trail on the right. The Stinger is a popular mountain biking access trail to the TRT, and the trail builders have taken this into account by adding mountain biking features, including flattened logs to roll onto and ride along and several rock jumps, on this section of TRT.

The TRT soon reaches an open area with sage and chinquapin before rolling up and down to an intersection with the Castle

> **SIDE TRIP Sierra Canyon Trail**
>
> The Sierra Canyon Trail drops 3500 feet in 9.6 miles to Genoa, Nevada's oldest town. Completed in 2011, the SCT connects the Carson Valley with the Tahoe Rim Trail. In case you missed that, I said 3500 feet, which is a lot of elevation gain or drop. This is not a Sunday stroll. The good news is that they built in a lot of switchbacks to ease the burden and the views of the Carson Valley are excellent.

Rock Vista Trail, on your right, 0.5 mile past the Stinger Trail (see side trip "Castle Rock Vista").

The TRT heads downhill for 0.1 mile where it meets the Castle Rock Road Trail, upon which a half-mile walk brings you to Andria Drive near the Kingsbury North Trailhead. If you start at the Castle Rock Road Trail, you can reach the top of the Castle Rock Trail in a mile of walking.

SIDE TRIP **Castle Rock Vista**

The trail climbs up 0.4 mile moderately steeply through lupine and pinemat manzanita to the top of this very interesting rock formation. Primarily built by the Boy Scouts, the trail winds through a rock chasm to reach the narrow top, where the views of much of the lake and South Lake Tahoe make this side jaunt well worth the effort.

As the TRT descends again, you pass huge granite boulders and walk into the cleavage between two rounded mounds. After passing a view of Castle Rock, the trail meets another junction, where a short use trail takes you to Mary Anne Drive, whose houses you can see clearly through the woods. Now walking through these Kingsbury neighborhoods, prime dog-walking terrain, you gently climb through fabulous rock formations between the two knobs. A path through the rocks leads to the Grubb viewpoint, where you find nice flat rocks and panoramic views of the lake. Just past the viewpoint is a 100-foot-long section; it took a crew of trail builders five weeks just to move all the car-sized boulders to provide a smooth surface for this little section of trail. We are talking world class trail building here, folks.

Your trail descends through the rocks to a grove of aspens and a dirt road that the trail follows for a short distance to a usually dry creek crossing. In the spring if you do find water here, it will be the first source since Marlette Campground, but there is a better source only about a mile farther. You head away from the aspens uphill to a junction, 2.7 miles from the junction with the Kingsbury North Access Trail and 1.3 miles from Mary Anne Drive. Here you turn left if you would like to hike the 6.7-mile North Daggett Loop (see side trip, next page).

SIDE TRIP **North Daggett Loop Trail**

From the junction with the TRT, the North Daggett Loop Trail climbs up 0.25 mile to North Benjamin Drive. The trail then climbs across a manzanita-covered slope to views of the lake. Just 0.4 mile from North Benjamin, you meet the North Daggett Summit Connector Trail. Here a right turn takes you 0.2 mile to the top of Kingsbury Grade, where you can cross the busy road to Tramway, which you can follow past the Tramway Market, 1.5 miles to the Stagecoach parking lot and the Kingsbury South TRT Trailhead.

On the loop trail you veer left, go gently downhill, and cross over to the Carson Valley side of the ridge, where a steady climb up a warm, dry slope awaits. Then, back on the Tahoe side of the ridge, your trail follows an old dirt road. At 1.8 miles from the North Benjamin and Andria crossing you reach a junction near a saddle, where a left turn takes you to a pleasant lake view vista in 0.2 mile.

Past the vista junction, the North Daggett Loop Trail descends for 0.4 mile to Donna/Kimberly Brooke Road, where you traverse up through manzanita, pass through a dry meadow, and top out on a ridge with views of houses below and the lake in the distance. At 3.5 miles from the southbound TRT, you reach Andria Drive, across the street from the Kingsbury North Trailhead. Congratulations, you have completed the 6.7-mile TRT and North Daggett Loop Trail.

The TRT goes just another 0.2 mile to the Kingsbury Grade crossing by traversing a slope and topping a small ridge, before a short, steep descent brings you to the highway. Carefully and swiftly cross this busy, windy road with little sight distance, and parallel Buchanan Road, which has an alternative access point behind a Forest Service gate, but without parking.

On the TRT an easy descent from the initial climb brings you through open forest to Edgewood Creek Road. You follow this lightly used dirt road 0.4 mile along the riparian zone of unseen Edgewood Creek, until at a sharp right turn you leave the road and cross year-round Edgewood Creek. This is the first reliable source of water for southbound TRT hikers since Marlette Campground, 26 miles north. With views of nearby homes and Mt. Tallac, the trail crests a ridge and then starts downhill through a boulder field. Stop to enjoy the best lake views since crossing Kingbury Grade and to get ready for an uphill that is coming soon.

A sharp downhill takes you under electric lines and a crossing of another branch of Edgewood Creek before the beginning of a steady climb through thick forest up a north-facing slope, which holds the snow longer than the rest of this section of trail. While you are climbing in earnest, there are frequent breaks and well-placed switchbacks to ease the burden. Deer are frequently seen, as are bike riders and neighborhood dog walkers. You pass some ancient western white pines until you meet a junction at 2.3 miles from Kingsbury Grade, at the top of a series of long switchbacks. A left turn takes you in 0.1 mile to the Brisack Viewpoint, where you find a good swath of big blue.

Back on the TRT, just 0.3 mile past the vista junction, you reach the Van Sickle Trail junction at the top of the saddle immediately before entering Heavenly Ski Resort lands (see side trip "Van Sickle Trail").

From this junction, a long gentle traverse takes you to the top of a swale, with a ski run on your left and a chairlift below it. You cross over the ski run to the forested slope and pass underneath the North Bowl chairlift. You soon meet a major ski run (dirt road) right at a hairpin turn in the road. The junction can be confusing; look for the TRT to the right and slightly uphill from

SIDE TRIP Van Sickle Trail

The combination TRT and Van Sickle Bi-State Park Trail is a wonderful new addition to the TRT trail network completed in 2012. In 3 miles TRT hikers can walk to the heart of the casino area in South Lake Tahoe.

The trail starts out as a mile-long west-heading traverse on a steep north-facing slope, with occasional, but nothing fancy glimpses of the lakes and the mountains to the north. Then the trail comes around the slope of the ridge and voilà, the whole world unfolds before you. The next mile you pass spectacular lake views and creek crossings, before walking right through the middle of the burn zone of the Gondola Fire to a waterfall 2.2 miles from the TRT junction. The incredible views continue, and the crowds increase during the last mile down through open slopes to the Van Sickle Bi-State Park.

Located right on the California and Nevada state line, the entrance to the park is only a hundred yards from Heavenly Village with supermarkets, restaurants, cinemas, and casinos. Thru-hikers looking for a quick return to civilization or a reminder of why they went into the woods in the first place would enjoy this trail halfway through their two-week adventure. In addition, bus service is available from the Visitor Center in Stateline to the Kingsbury South Trailhead.

Looking toward Emerald Bay from South Camp Peak

the turn of the road. Do *not* follow the road as it goes off to the left and downhill.

Another third of a mile on the trail takes you under the Stagecoach chairlift and then to the Stagecoach ski run, which you cross to meet the original TRT route and the end of this section. Thru-hikers continue straight ahead. The TRT Kingsbury South Trailhead is now accessed with a left turn, which takes you downhill moderately steeply, through thick brush and trees, around a condo development, to the trailhead in the Stagecoach parking lot in about a half mile.

SECTION 5

Kingsbury Grade to Big Meadow

(23.2 miles)

Difficulty This long and relatively strenuous section has a lot of elevation changes and a 9730-foot high point. While this trail is too long for many to hike in one day, for the strong hiker it is a wonderful dayhike.

Best Seasons Each end of the trail can be hiked as early as mid-June. The highest part of the trail near Freel Peak is usually not open until mid-July or later, depending upon the amount of snow that fell the previous winter. The first major snows at Freel Peak may come as early as the middle of October.

Highlights This trail section provides tremendous views of Lake Tahoe, Carson Valley, Desolation Wilderness, and the Carson Range. In addition, it has a wonderful high-elevation lake, Star Lake, and access to the summit of the two highest peaks in the Tahoe Basin: Freel (10,881 feet) and Jobs Sister (10,823 feet).

Heads Up! Some sections of the trail are above 9000 feet, and much of the trail is open and exposed to the sun and wind—*bring your sunscreen.* As with all sections of the trail along the east shore of Lake Tahoe, water is in short supply. In the first few miles out from the Stagecoach parking lot, there are several seasonal streams, with the South Fork of Daggett Creek lasting the longest. Star Lake, which you will reach 8.8 miles from the Kingsbury Trailhead, is a delightful swimming spot, but its high silt content may clog your filter. Better drinking water is available about 1 mile past Star Lake where you find the lovely, swift-moving Cold Creek, fresh from the slopes of Freel Peak. On slopes west of Freel Peak, several small streams cascade across the trail into late summer.

From Armstrong Pass you may find water by heading southeast from the TRT on the steep Armstrong Pass connector trail.

LAKE TAHOE

It is 0.4 mile long, and near its bottom you cross a small stream. From its trailhead a dirt road descends almost 0.5 mile to cross larger Willow Creek. You can find reliable water just below the west edge of the western Freel Meadow. Finally, east of the Big Meadow Trailhead, there is Grass Lake Creek, a major stream, at approximately 0.5 mile, and another one 2 miles from the trailhead at the Grass Lake Trail junction.

As with the entire East Shore, the amount of water in creeks varies tremendously from year to year. I have seen Mott Canyon Creek roar in September and be dry as a bone in August. Always take into account how much it snowed in the area the previous winter when making water plans. If you don't know what sort of winter it was, ask any Tahoe local, but be prepared for a animated and detailed explanation.

Tips for Mountain Bikers This section is challenging, loved by some and hated by others. It has lots of technical areas with hundreds of rock benches that will require many riders to dismount. Portions of the trail are along steep drops that may unnerve some riders. The first portion is primarily a long steady climb, with the exception of a brief steep downhill on some very sandy, loose soil. Once you get to the top of Monument Pass, just about when you are wondering why you are doing this, the trail levels off a bit before some more climbing for several miles to Star Lake. After Star Lake it is a major, difficult climb again up to 9700 feet. Almost all the mountain bikers will be walking near the top. From the saddle of Freel Peak, it is time for a big downhill with a few tight switchbacks that may scare some riders.

Eventually, you reach Armstrong Pass, a great place to escape if you have had enough. A short trail descends to a dirt road, Forest Route 051F, that you can follow 0.5 mile down to Forest Route 051; take it 3.5 miles to Highway 89. If you do this, you will reach Highway 89 about 0.8 mile east of signed Luther Pass and 1.8 miles above the Highway 88 and 89 junction in Hope Valley. If you continue toward Big Meadow, you will confront another long uphill, followed by another long downhill.

SIDE TRIP **Mr. Toad's Wild Ride**

This popular mountain biking trail is usually accessed via the Big Meadow Trailhead and is known as Mr. Toad's Wild Ride. If you start at Big Meadow, this ride starts with a long uphill followed by a big challenging downhill. Before you ride this section, read the mountain biking tips at the beginning of this section. This trail is recommended for expert riders only.

Along the downhill section, you pass the junction to the Saxon Creek Trail. This very popular mountain biking trail, usually accessed via the Big Meadow Trailhead, is known as Mr. Toad's Wild Ride. While some may find it a wild ride, I found it to be very chewed up, steep, and impossible to navigate in many sections. If you go, be prepared for difficulty. Past it is a brief steep uphill, followed by a steady downhill to the end of the trail, which is fun, but still has several technically challenging sections.

Getting There, Kingsbury South Trailhead to Big Meadow Trailhead From Stateline in the South Lake Tahoe area, drive east up Highway 207 (Kingsbury Grade) 3.2 miles to Tramway Drive at Daggett Pass, the summit of Kingsbury Grade. Follow the signs 1.5 miles to the Heavenly Valley Resort Stagecoach parking lot.

Getting There, Big Meadow Trailhead to Kingsbury South Trailhead From the intersection of Highway 89 and Highway 50 in Meyers, drive 5.3 miles south on Highway 89 to the Big Meadow Trailhead and parking area on your left. Luther Pass is 3.3 miles farther. This trail can also be accessed from the Grass Lake Trailhead, which you will find by driving south on Highway 89 past the Big Meadow Trailhead for 1.5 miles. Park on the right side of the road in a roadside pullout, and cross the highway to the trail. If you pass Grass Lake, the lake that looks like a meadow on the right, you have gone too far.

Trail Description

Amid high-rise condominiums and a huge parking lot, the trailhead is located near a ski lift. Are we talking a wilderness experi-

Big Meadow

ence here or what? Don't worry—it gets better. You start with a steep 0.4-mile climb through thick brush and forest on this TRT access trail to a junction with the main TRT. Here, a right turn takes you across a ski run and toward the Van Sickle Trail and Kingsbury North. Your route is left, where the trail switchbacks moderately up through a forest of red firs and Jeffrey pines and provides views of the condos below and later brief glimpses of Lake Tahoe and Washoe Valley. You walk over numerous granite boulders and steps, which are challenging to those on bikes.

After climbing for close to 1 mile you reach a saddle and then descend gently for 0.5 mile, passing under another Heavenly Resort ski lift. In another 130 yards you cross the South Fork of Daggett Creek, which runs most of the year. It provides a patch of greenery and wildflowers in this land of ski runs. As you ascend again, western white pines and lodgepole pines replace the red firs and Jeffrey pines.

Next the trail gently climbs through alternating areas of dense forest and a more open combination of brush and forest with manzanita and tobacco brush dominating the scene. The open vegetation allows views east to Carson Valley and the desert ranges beyond it. About 0.75 mile past the creek you reach the north rim of Mott Canyon, where you see Freel Peak. You follow the rim for a moderate 0.5-mile ascent west, then climb gently 0.25 mile south to where, about 3.3 miles from the trailhead, you reach a saddle and a ski area maintenance road. You drop very steeply, on this road over soft, sandy soil (careful on your bike!) into Mott Canyon. If you think this short section is steep going down, put on a backpack and hike up it. It's enough to make you want to hike clockwise. Just underneath the Mott Canyon chairlift is beautiful little Mott Canyon Creek. In the early summer, its banks are covered with Lewis's monkeyflower, yellow monkeyflower, delphinium, and columbine. The lovely stream runs most of the season, but may dry up by fall.

After a short distance with a moderate climb, you come out of Mott Canyon and round the corner to an open traverse. Your route is now mostly treeless and facing east with stunning views of Carson Valley far below to the east and Jobs Sister, with its huge drop in elevation from mountaintop to valley floor, in the distance to the south. To your left, steeply below, is evidence of a major forest fire reaching up toward Jobs Sister from the Carson Valley. Here you will see mountain mahogany and the largest western white pine I have ever come upon just to the left side of the trail. With a circumference of 24 feet, the pine provides shade in this hot, exposed section of trail. While it is beautiful to hike, anyone who is afraid of heights will find this cliff-edge section of trail a challenging bike ride, which becomes steeper toward Monument Pass.

Approximately 5 miles from the trailhead, you climb to Monument Pass, which is crossed by powerlines and is about 0.4 mile beyond the Nevada-California boundary. At the pass you cross from the Carson side (eastern slope) to the Tahoe side on the western slope. Monument Peak at higher than 10,000 feet is a towering presence to the west. Dramatic views of Jobs Sister and Freel Peak immediately open up. Here you reach a junction with the Monument Pass to High Meadows Trail (see side trip "Monument Pass to High Meadows").

On the TRT it is 3.7 miles from Monument Pass to Star Lake. The first 2 miles are on a gentle, sandy path through mostly open terrain, and provide a wonderful opportunity to marvel at the views of Desolation Wilderness, including Pyramid Peak, the Crystal Range, and Lake Tahoe to the west. The results of the Angora Fire come clearly into view. This fire in the summer of 2007 burned more than 3,000 acres and 250 homes near South Lake Tahoe. As you get closer to Star Lake, the immense size of the Freel Peak massif becomes more and more impressive. A little more than 1 mile before Star Lake, the trail begins to ascend again, sometimes moderately, and the tree cover of western white pine, lodgepole, and hemlock gets thicker.

Finally you reach Star Lake, located at the base of Jobs Sister, which rises dramatically from its shores. This alluring lake will take your breath away, especially if you venture into its cold waters (although after an extended warm period the water temperatures can become quite bearable). As the only large lake on the Tahoe Rim Trail between Mt. Rose and Luther Pass, it may be the best place for those who are doing an overnight trip to set up camp. There are several overused camping spots close to the lake and lots of wonderful camping spots above the lake. The Star Lake to High Meadows Trail, completed in 2012, descends 1500 feet in 4.5 miles, to High Meadows, where an additional 3 miles on the Cold Creek Trail will bring you to the High Meadows Trailhead.

When you leave Star Lake, the trail can be a bit confusing and challenging; just follow the rocky pathway over the lake's outlet. I find the first mile or so after Star Lake the most interesting mile of this section of the TRT. You begin with a moderate climb from

> **SIDE TRIP Monument Pass to High Meadows**
>
> This beautiful trail drops more than 1000 feet in 3 miles through unique rock formations and groves of aspens to High Meadows. At High Meadows you can catch the Cold Creek Trail and in an additional 3 miles reach the High Meadows Trailhead. You can also hike a loop by taking the High Meadows to Star Lake Trail, which heads uphill 1500 feet in 4.5 miles to the shores of Star Lake. Are you spending a layover day at Star Lake? Then perhaps this 11-mile loop will make an afternoon swim in Star's chilly waters especially attractive.

Star Lake with good views of Lake Tahoe. You are now in the wide open at a high altitude where western white pines, whitebark pines, and hemlocks are scattered among the sandy soil. Many of the trees have been tortured by high-altitude winds and are stunted and bent. You also see numerous large pieces of white quartz along this section as well as patches of snow that hang on late into the summer. You head steadily toward 10,000 feet, passing an early summer waterfall and then viewing the imposing hulk of Freel Peak.

You will arrive at a swiftly moving, clear mountain stream, a tributary of Cold Creek. Only a foot or two wide, it creates a green grassy path through the desolate sand and rock. If you head upstream, you will find open terrain, good for camping. This is an excellent water source. As you reach the saddle below Freel Peak, at the high point of 9730 feet, don't be surprised to find a patch of snow even in late July. This often windswept spot is about 1.9 miles south of Star Lake and 3.0 miles north of Armstrong Pass (see side trip "Freel Peak").

Those who find more than 23 miles just about enough to hike can skip Freel Peak and continue on the TRT. Here you are almost midway through Section 5, about 10.8 miles south of the Kingsbury South Trailhead, and about 12.5 miles north of the Big Meadow Trailhead. Your trail begins with a long, steady, thinly forested descent 0.7 mile south to a switchback, which turns you back to the north. You continue downhill for an additional 0.3 mile before switching back again to the south. Once again, you will enjoy excellent views of the Crystal Range, the massive granite ridge on the western edge of Desolation Wilderness. You soon cross three spring-fed creeks that

---

SIDE TRIP Freel Peak

At this saddle, you can begin a steep climb to the top of Freel Peak, at 10,881 feet the tallest peak on the Tahoe Basin rim. The trail switchbacks up the steep slope, climbing 1150 feet in elevation in a mile to the top of the peak. From Freel Peak you can easily hike cross-country over to the top of Jobs Sister (10,823 feet). Climbing these peaks makes for challenging, but beautiful jaunts if you are camping in the Star Lake area, and of course the views are spectacular.

are usually flowing and provide much-needed water and beautiful wildflower displays. These little ribbons of color in this dry, brown landscape are a welcome relief. Less than 0.5 mile past the last streamlet is a huge mass of granite with a steep cliff face and lots of fascinating rock formations known as Fountain Face, about 1 mile north of Armstrong Pass.

Less than 0.3 mile before Armstrong Pass, the trail is gently graded; you experience a gentle up-and-down traverse and pass many large juniper trees, with their light blue berries and gnarled trunks and branches, along the way.

At the deep crest notch of Armstrong Pass, you can leave the TRT to shorten your hike. (Or, if you come in from Armstrong Pass, it makes for a relatively short way to access Freel Peak.) The short, steep Armstrong Pass Trail takes you 0.4 mile to an old abandoned road. Follow this road 0.5 mile to trailhead parking just across a small bridge. From here it is 3.4 miles to Highway 89 and about 5 miles to Hope Valley. Follow the Armstrong Pass Trailhead directions below in reverse (see side trip "Armstrong Pass," next page).

A Tale of Two Fountains

The Fountain Place you see on the map is a meadow area, below to the west. Both Fountain Face and Fountain Place were named for Garret Fountain, who built a way station at Fountain Place in 1860 in an effort to supply miners on their way from California to the Comstock Lode in Nevada. Fountain hoped they would go over Armstrong Pass, but instead they chose Daggett Pass, and his dream failed.

The Armstrong Pass junction is located at the top of the U-shaped valley at the end of the long southward traverse. Here, the trail rounds a corner of the ridge and heads west. From Armstrong Pass, the journey to Big Meadow is 9.5 miles. In just 0.1 mile you reach a junction with a trail that descends northwest toward Fountain Place and Oneidas Street. This trail is another access to the TRT from South Lake Tahoe. The TRT quickly leaves the ridge to begin this next phase with a steady, sometimes steep uphill climb on sandy soils through a forest of scattered western white pine, lodgepole pine, and red fir. Your views are now fewer and less dramatic with occasional glimpses of the Freel massif to your northeast as you switchback up the ridgeline past some large trees.

The area between Big Meadow and Armstrong Pass is popular for mountain biking. If you are on your bike, enjoy, but watch out for hikers. Be a little more vigilant if you are hiking. While portions of this section are a fun sandy ride, there are a lot of short rocky sections that will force many riders to get off their bikes; other sections are composed of deep granite gravel that will make it tough, whether you are going up or down. After 2 miles of switchbacking uphill, you reach an open, broad ridge with large boulders and views to the south of numerous peaks above 10,000 feet, including Round Top near Carson Pass at 10,381 feet.

The trail soon leaves the ridge and proceeds through a rocky area with stone steps, then it continues through an open forest until, at a little less than 3 miles from Armstrong Pass, you traverse the largest of three meadows known as Freel Meadows. USGS maps show this area as Freel Meadows, but they are not specific about how many meadows are included. When I scouted the area, I found three meadowlike areas within 1.5 miles. The first meadow is a mostly treeless slope dotted with

SIDE TRIP **Armstrong Pass**

To access Armstrong Pass from Highway 89 (a section of road recommended only for 4-wheel-drive vehicles with high clearance), take Highway 89 south from its junction with Highway 50 in Meyers up to signed Luther Pass, just beyond a large grassy meadow holding Grass Lake. Start on a long downhill toward Hope Valley going 0.8 mile to a junction with Forest Service Road 051 on your left. Watch closely and slow down; it is easy to miss. (This junction is 1.8 miles up from the Highway 88 junction down in Hope Valley.) Take this road steeply uphill. In 1.1 miles the road divides. There is a gate on the right fork, but stay left. At 1.6 miles, bear left. At 1.8 miles, you cross a cattle guard and then continue to bear left.

At 2.4 miles, you reach your first bridge as you follow a stream. At 2.7 miles, at a fork in the road, go straight ahead. At 3.4 miles, you will reach the second bridge; cross this bridge, then immediately make a 180-degree left turn into a small parking area. Park here and then walk across a trail bridge and go 0.5 mile uphill on the now abandoned road to the Armstrong Pass connector trail. Take this trail 0.4 mile steeply uphill to the junction with the TRT.

Freel Peak

mules ears, lupine, and paintbrush, (the actual meadow lies at the base of the slopes). There are beautiful Sierra peaks visible to the south. Just past the open slopes, you reach an excellent viewpoint to the north. Here you see deep, boggy Hell Hole Canyon directly below you, and farther in the distance to the north, Lake Tahoe. To the northeast, Freel Peak stands out in full relief. I dry camped here once and found that it was the perfect spot to enjoy a sunset. Next, you pass through an open forest before reaching a large grassy meadow to your left (the second meadow). Then shortly you reach a third meadow, this one loaded with wildflowers, including corn lily, lupine, and delphinium. You can get water from the west end of this meadow at the headwaters of Saxon Creek. The Freel Meadows area is a wonderful green divide between the more barren sandy slopes of the higher elevations to the east and the thick forest that appears after the meadows.

After leaving this meadow, you descend at a moderate pace through denser forest. About 1 mile later and 5.1 miles from Armstrong Pass, you reach the Saxon Creek Trail (alias "Mr. Toad's Wild Ride") on a broad saddle just above Tucker Flat.

Star Lake

With 4.4 miles left, you continue on the TRT over a short uphill section northwest, followed by a short traverse west, and then you meander downhill 2 miles through primarily dense forest of red and white firs and western white and Jeffrey pines to the Grass Lake Trail. Along the way you see several small meadows with many wildflowers, especially mules ears. There are also two viewing spots. The first is near the top on a very short use trail to a rock outcropping with views to the northwest of Lake Tahoe. The second viewpoint is after the trail switchbacks down through the forest to another rock outcropping on the east side of the ridge. Here you have views of the mountains to the east and southeast. A small creek, shaded by lush aspen trees, that you cross pops out of a jumble of huge granite boulders and makes for a special visual treat.

At 2.0 miles from the Big Meadow Trailhead, you meet the Grass Lake Trail, an alternative TRT route to Highway 89. On the Grass Lake Trail, you can hike only 0.6 mile to meet Highway 89, which is 1.4 miles shorter if you are walking or riding (and 400 feet less climbing and descending) than on the trail to the Big Meadows Trailhead. If you are heading to the Grass Lake Trailhead, you will find a moderately steep downhill through the trees to the trailhead located next to Highway 89. You have now had the pleasure of being on the first section of the Tahoe Rim Trail, which was built by the Tahoe Rim Trail Association in 1984.

There is a small but reliable stream near the junction of the Grass Lake connector and the Tahoe Rim Trail. There is only one more water source, Grass Lake Creek, in the next 1.6 miles, about 0.4 mile from the end of the trail. It is a larger stream and a good water source. If you continue to the Big Meadow Trailhead, you will journey through more of the same terrain, a gentle downhill on many switchbacks through a mostly thick forest of predominantly Jeffrey pine and red fir. While you cannot see Highway 89 from the trail, you can often hear it.

At the finish, you arrive at a paved road, on which you turn left and go 100 yards to the entrance to a large parking lot and restroom facility (which has no water). At this junction you can turn right and find an overflow campground with toilet, trash receptacles, food storage lockers, and tent sites only 0.25 mile down the paved road. The next section of the TRT heads up to Big Meadow, Round Lake, and eventually the Pacific Crest Trail; it is past the trailhead restrooms at the southwest corner of the parking lot.

SECTION 6

Big Meadow Trailhead to Echo Summit and Echo Lake

(15.3 miles to Echo Summit, 17.5 miles to Echo Lake)

Difficulty This section is moderately strenuous. Most of the trail is gentle up-and-down terrain or almost level through meadows or open fields. While there are several sustained climbs, they are not too steep, and most people will not find this section of the TRT exceptionally difficult. The most difficult portion of the trail is between Bryan Meadow and Benwood Meadow, where you will experience an almost continuous, steep descent (or a steep climb if you are coming from Echo Summit, especially with a backpack).

Best Seasons This section of trail is best hiked from late June to early October. While you may see a few snow patches well into July, the trail is mostly snow-free by late June. The wildflowers come into full bloom in late July or early August, which makes that the best time to hike this section. When those flowers are in bloom, you are in for an incredible treat.

Highlights There are three beautiful lakes on this trip: Round Lake is only a 5.2-mile round-trip from the trailhead. Dardanelles is 1.4 miles off the TRT and provides a 6.8-mile round-trip. Showers Lake is a good halfway stop 7 miles into the 15-mile hike. You will find impressive volcanic rock formations jutting high above the shores of Round Lake and on the ridges above Meiss Meadows. There are two large meadows, Big Meadow and Meiss Meadows, which, if you come at the right time of year, will provide you with some of the most stunning displays of wildflowers you will see on the Rim Trail. In addition, the trail has other interesting flora, including some spectacular juniper trees. In a wonderful large bowl just past Showers Lake, you will encounter waterfalls and numerous wildflower-bordered streams caused

by springtime snowmelt, as well as spectacular castlelike volcanic rock formations. This section may have the greatest variety of views and habitats of any section of the TRT.

Heads Up! While the trail has several good water sources and places to swim, the second half of the trail, between Showers Lake and Echo Summit, has more limited water supplies, especially in the fall. Water can be found at the following locations: About 0.7 mile south of the Big Meadow Trailhead you will find Big Meadow Creek, which may dry up in the fall, at the edge of Big Meadow. The Upper Truckee River in Meiss Meadows is a major swift-flowing stream. About halfway through the hike is Showers Lake, an excellent water source. Less than a mile past Showers Lake you will find several streams cascading down from the lava flows above. Just before reaching Benwood Meadow you will cross a small stream that is usually flowing.

The 2 miles of the trail descending to Benwood Meadow are quite steep, which can be very hard on the knees and every other body part. From the Echo Summit end, this is a major uphill starting just 1 mile into your hike.

Tips for Mountain Bikers From the Big Meadow Trailhead bikes are allowed on the first 5 miles to the junction of the Tahoe Rim Trail and the Pacific Crest Trail. Bikes are *not* allowed on the Pacific Crest Trail, so this ride is a 10-mile out-and-back. Much of this ride is technically challenging, with lots of rocks, but for experienced riders it can be a fun ride.

Getting There, Big Meadow to Echo Summit From the intersection of Highways 89 and 50 in Meyers (south of South Lake Tahoe), drive 5.3 miles south on Highway 89 to the Big Meadow Trailhead on your left (this is about 3.3 miles before signed Luther Pass). The previous segment from Kingsbury Grade to Big Meadow Trailhead ends here, and you start across the road and head uphill toward Big Meadow. The trailhead has a restroom facility and information kiosks.

Showers Lake

Getting There, Echo Summit to Big Meadow Drive west on Highway 50 from South Lake Tahoe to the top of Echo Summit (4 miles west of the intersection of Highways 89 and 50 in Meyers). Just 0.3 mile past Echo Summit, make a left turn, which is marked with an Echo Summit Sno-Park sign. Park on the southern end of the parking lot, and find the trail just to the west.

Trail Description

The trail starts out at the lowest point in the Big Meadow Trailhead parking lot (southwest end). You walk about 250 yards through a forest of white fir, Jeffrey pine, and juniper before you cross Highway 89. Once you cross the road the trail starts south. It is moderately steep, taking you uphill over rocky terrain through a thicker forest of Jeffrey pine, western white pine, and fir. After a little more than 0.2 mile you pass to the left of Big Meadow Creek, whose bed is filled with huge granite boulders and lined with aspen trees. By 0.3 mile from the trailhead the grade moderates, becoming almost level as you walk close to a stream on the right surrounded in the fall by the yellow leaves of aspen trees.

Stop and shut your eyes and listen to the quaking sound that gives the aspen its name.

Soon you reach a junction. A left turn here would take you to Scotts Lake. Your trail, however, continues straight ahead to a large flat meadow with the new and original name of "Big Meadow." Just as you enter the meadow, the trail crosses a stream, which is good-sized in the spring, but may dry up in late summer. This is, of course, Big Meadow Creek. As you head south across the meadow, you are treated to views of the surrounding mountains to your southwest. At only 0.7 mile from the trailhead, you can reach the meadow in half an hour and enjoy a wonderful setting.

After you cross the meadow, the trail heads uphill again through the fairly dense forest of lodgepole, western white pine, and red fir. The tree cover thins out as you reach more open and sunny areas with sagebrush and a variety of wildflowers including lupine, mules ears, and pennyroyal. You now occasionally pass small groves of aspen trees. About 1 mile past the meadow you reach a saddle, and head 0.25 mile downhill on steep trail that affords you great mountain views to the south and west. At 2 miles from the trailhead you reach a junction. To your right, the Meiss Meadows Trail (Christmas Valley on the sign) will take you toward Dardanelles Lake in 1.4 miles (see side trip "Dardanelles Lake").

> ### SIDE TRIP Dardanelles Lake
>
> To reach Dardanelles Lake, you descend northwest on the Meiss Meadows Trail for 0.2 mile through a mixed forest of pine, fir, and a few junipers to another trail which you take; you will hike an additional 1.2 miles on it to Dardanelles Lake. The trail first crosses a creek and then levels off in a grassy meadow before it climbs again up a rocky tread. You reach Dardanelles Lake on a big granite flat that overlooks the lake.
>
> Above the lake's south shore is a massive rock cliff reaching right down to the water. There are great camping spots at Dardanelles Lake above a large flat expanse of granite that reaches down to the northeast shore of the lake. The midsummer water can be warm in this beautiful lake, so enjoy a swim and then bask on the granite slab. Ah . . . now you know why you put that backpack on. Be forewarned, however; since the lake is only 3.4 miles from the trailhead, you are not likely to be swimming alone.

On the TRT you continue straight ahead and begin a gentle ascent through some very interesting volcanic rock mudflow formations. At 2.6 miles from the trailhead (and 0.6 mile from the last junction), you reach the northeast corner of Round Lake. Round Lake is the largest lake you will encounter on this section of trail and offers great swimming and camping. The best campsite is at the lake's northwest corner by the outlet, but the lake can get crowded on a sunny summer weekend. Thanks to an influx of volcanic sediments, Round Lake's color varies from a brownish-green to an unusual aqua-blue, more reminiscent of the lakes and streams of western Canada than most of the lakes in the Sierra. As you walk past Round Lake, a spectacular steep cliff of volcanic rock reaches skyward on your left. You will have the pleasure of gazing at this fascinating rock formation, known as the Dardanelles, from several locations as you complete your hike.

Just after Round Lake you pass a small seasonal stream and lush meadow area with willows and wildflowers, including lupine, monkshood, Lewis's monkeyflower, paintbrush, ranger's buttons, and groundsel. You then ascend to an open area with aspen and sagebrush that provides views of the volcanic ridgeline to your west. The next 0.5 mile or so is a pleasant, mostly level walk through wildflowers and scattered aspen groves quaking in the wind. Beautiful mountain views are available in every direction. You begin a gentle ascent into a forest of scattered conifers and then head downhill again past a luscious meadow with more mountain views before you reach the Pacific Crest Trail 4.9 miles from your trailhead. Across the large open meadow, you will see a charming old cowboy cabin, once the home of the Meiss family, whom the meadows were named after; they lived here while grazing their cattle. While you cannot enter the cabins, a use trail leads to an information plaque next to them.

You have now reached the Pacific Crest Trail (PCT), which travels from Canada to Mexico. If Mexico is your goal, turn left, and in a few months you will be there on the PCT. If you would prefer heading up to Canada, turn right. Either way, it's a long trip. This junction is located at the southernmost point of the Tahoe Rim Trail, and as you turn right at the junction, you begin heading north. For about the next 50 miles the PCT and TRT are one trail. In addition to the Pacific Crest Trail and the Tahoe Rim Trail, your footpath is now also a part of the little-used Tahoe-Yosemite Trail (TYT), which travels from Tuolumne Meadows in Yosemite to Meeks Bay on the west shore of Lake Tahoe, a distance of a little more than 185 miles. The PCT, TRT, and TYT are one trail for the next 29 miles, until the TYT heads over Phipps Pass, past a chain of lakes known as the Tallant Lakes, down to Meeks Bay.

You turn right at this junction and begin your journey northwest with a lovely walk up the long valley of the Upper Truckee River. With high volcanic ridges to the east and west and a beautiful almost-level valley floor seasonally filled with wildflowers to walk across, it can be a highlight of your day. The flowers will vary from year to year, but you can expect to see low-lying lupine and elephant heads in prolific display. As you walk northwest for about 0.5 mile on the PCT, you can see Meiss Lake across 0.5 mile of swampy meadow to the north. This very shallow, warm lake makes a pleasant swimming hole in late summer. During the early summer, the walk to the lake is swampy, and you may lose blood to mosquitoes.

Mostly through the meadow you meet the Upper Truckee River, a good source for water or for catching your breath, but a potentially wet ford in early summer. After 1.5 miles through the meadow, a fairly steep climb awaits you for the last 0.5 mile up to Showers Lake. This steady uphill push through a mixture of deep forest and open fields gives you prolific displays of tall lupine, fireweed, and paintbrush. As you rise, you are rewarded with glorious views to the south and east of Meiss Meadows and the Dardanelles.

Just before you reach the shores of Showers Lake, a trail on your left heads steeply up to the ridge above the lake. It leads to Schneider Cow Camp but also provides access to awe-inspiring

Castle formations north of Showers Lake

views of the whole of Meiss Meadows, and if you follow the flat ridgetop away from the trail, views of Showers Lake far below.

Showers Lake itself is beautiful. The south side is marshy, but the northern side provides great swimming opportunities enhanced by flat granite rocks that reach down to the water. There are several camping spots surrounded by hemlock, lodgepole pines, and before late summer, mosquitoes, above the north and east sides of the lake. Unfortunately all that goodness comes with a price. This might be the most popular place to camp on the Tahoe Rim Trail.

To continue past Showers Lake, your trail first heads steeply down below the lake's outlet and then climbs back up on the other side of the outlet's gully. You head for the next 0.5 mile through a pleasant forest with scattered trees and a few wildflower-dotted meadows until you reach the edge of an enormous bowl. This 0.7-mile-wide bowl is a beautiful mixture of castle-shaped volcanic rock formations, little streams plunging down steep, rocky gullies, thick fields of lupine and paintbrush, and sometimes even late season snowfields. Several swiftly moving cascades and stunning views to the east of Lake Tahoe, Dardanelles Lake, and Freel

Peak complete this idyllic picture. It is a gentle climb across the bowl, and during midsummer the streams cascading down from the slopes above provide water for you and support an abundance of wildflowers. Near the end of the bowl, the path becomes steeper and the terrain, drier, until you reach a minor saddle on a crest where the surroundings change. Now you enter an area with sandy soils and scattered trees; mostly western white pine, lodgepole pine, and hemlock.

First you climb slowly, and then the trail levels off and soon reaches the Schneider Cow Camp Trail, which turns to your left and heads first west and then southwest. Now at 1.9 miles north of Showers Lake, you continue north and make a 0.2-mile moderate descent to a saddle with an unmarked trail. Past this saddle junction your broad crest trail continues through the open hemlock forest, making several minor ascents and descents before leveling off and passing several more small meadows. At 3.5 miles from Showers Lake (and 1.6 miles north of the Schneider Cow Camp Trail junction), you meet another saddle junction, where a faded marked trail (that appears to be in danger of disappearing altogether) leads to Sayles Canyon.

The TRT continues along the sandy crest, mostly devoid of views, until a nice view opens up to the northwest of Pyramid Peak, the tallest peak of the huge granite ridgeline known as the Crystal Range, which lies in the heart of Desolation Wilderness. If you are thru-hiking, you will get much closer views of the Crystal Range as you walk along Lake Aloha about 15 miles north of here, but first you must finish this section. At 4.4 miles from Showers Lake, you reach Bryan Meadow and the trail that leads to it, which is about 3.9 miles from the Echo Summit Trailhead (see side trip "Bryan Meadow Trail").

On the TRT just past the meadow you first descend briefly east to a minor gully and then climb, sometimes steeply, through a thick forest almost 0.5 mile to a ridge. After a steep uphill, what do you do next? Go downhill steeply of course, passing a rock outcropping just off the trail to the right. From here you can enjoy views of the Upper Truckee River Canyon, South Lake Tahoe Airport, and Lake Tahoe in the distance. Your trail quickly levels off, and you pass a pleasant little camping spot next to a small, usually reliable, stream in a flat area in the trees. This is one of the last good campsites before you reach Echo Summit.

Beyond it you begin a descent that starts out steep and becomes very steep as the trail heads down along the side of a granite ridge. The last time I walked this trail I found this downhill bone-jarring, toe-jamming, and knee-breaking—and those are just the words I can repeat! Since the first edition of this book, the TRTA has added several switchbacks easing the grade, but it is still very steep. The rocky descent is so steep at times that it becomes slippery, so watch your step. The trail follows the east ridge of a big granite canyon that ends at Benwood Meadow.

Take a few rest breaks to enjoy the beautiful granite rock formations and the especially large hem-

> **SIDE TRIP Bryan Meadow Trail**
>
> The Bryan Meadow Trail joins the Sayles Canyon Trail, and the combined trail descends an additional 0.6 mile to reach trailhead parking near the Sierra-at-Tahoe ski area. These trails provide another means to access Showers Lake for those in the Upper Highway 50 area. Bryan Meadow is a large, gently sloping meadow of grass and seasonal mud, but it has no apparent drinking water near the trail. However, you should find water about 0.5 mile down the Sayles Canyon Trail, at or just below the west end of the meadow.

locks you pass. Keep your eyes open for marmots since you are in their prime territory. Gazing across this deep canyon, you see a higher ridge of granite on the west side. You pass a massive juniper at a crest saddle, which provides a viewpoint to the south. Views are highlighted by the Dardanelles and Round Top, which holds its north-facing snowfields well into late summer. Eventually the downhill largely abates, after a grueling 2-mile descent, where you cross the canyon's stream on a wooden bridge and head into a lush shady area loaded with tiger lilies, thimbleberries, and ferns. Over the next 0.75 mile you continue on a gentle downhill with Benwood Meadow visible through the trees on your right.

Meiss Meadows

By the meadow's northeast edge, you reach a junction with an older trail coming from a little-used alternate trailhead. With only 0.75 mile remaining, turn left at the junction, and ascend gently north through a more open, drier forest of large Jeffrey pines and manzanita. A short distance before you reach the parking area, cross an old dirt road on a mostly treeless slope, formerly a ski area and now the winter location of Adventure Mountain Tahoe, a groomed sledding hill. Walk next to a parking lot to your car or Highway 50 and the next stretch of the Tahoe Rim Trail.

Echo Summit and Echo Lake to Barker Pass

(32.7 miles from Echo Lake, 34.7 miles from Echo Summit)

Difficulty This strenuous section has many ascents and descents. While other segments of the Rim Trail can be hiked or biked in a day, this trip requires at least two days (for most people), and I recommend three. It can also be completed in sections by hiking out to Fallen Leaf Lake on the Glen Alpine Trail or to Emerald Bay from either Dicks Lake or Middle Velma Lake via the Bay View Trail.

Best Seasons In a typical year, most of this section is snow-free from mid-July to late October. Sections of this trail, especially the area on the north side of Dicks Pass, may have patches of snow into August following heavy snow years.

Highlights A wonderful wilderness experience awaits you as you travel through the heart of Desolation Wilderness. You will pass or see many beautiful lakes, including Lower Echo, Upper Echo, Cagwin, Ralston, Tamarack, Aloha, Heather, Susie, Grass, Gilmore, Half Moon, Alta Morris, Dicks, Fontanillis, Upper Velma, Middle Velma, and Richardson. If you like to swim in mountain lakes, this is the trail for you. You will also cross a high mountain pass with incredible views into two enormous watersheds.

Heads Up! The starting elevation is about 7400 feet at Echo Lake, and you will rise to nearly 9400 feet at Dicks Pass. Water is plentiful for most of the trail, until you get north of Middle Velma Lake where the water sources between it and Richardson Lake can quickly decline. Beyond the latter, there are several streams and springs. The biggest year-round stream along this stretch is Miller Creek, located about 1.75 miles north of Richardson Lake. A few

Continued on p.159

Continued
on p.158

TRT thru-hikers near Susie Lake

miles farther gets you to Bear Creek. If you are thru-hiking, consider that north of Barker Pass it is another 2 miles before you reach water again.

You can cut off 2.5 miles of hiking by taking the Echo Lakes Water Taxi from the trailhead to Upper Echo Lake. The taxi only runs during the summer and when water is high enough for safe passage between Lower and Upper Echo Lakes. For information about the water taxi, call the Echo Lakes Chalet at (530) 659-7207.

It's beautiful, accessible, and very popular. If you want a true wilderness experience, Middle Velma Lake on a weekend in July is not the place to find it. Wilderness permits are required to enter Desolation Wilderness. Day-use permits are available at the trailhead. If you are camping, you must obtain a permit through the Forest Service. (Permit information can be found in Chapter 1, page 5.) The biggest concern with this section of trail, however, is that it is so magnificent you may want to stay forever, so be sure to bring along enough food.

Getting There, Echo to Barker This trail begins at either Echo Summit or Lower Echo Lake. Most people prefer to start at Lower

Echo Lake, where you can avoid 2.2 miles of mostly viewless hiking, much of it close to Highway 50 or among summer cabins.

Getting There, Echo Summit to Lower Echo Lake From Meyers take Highway 50 westbound to Echo Summit. From the summit, drive just 0.3 mile and turn left. You will see an Echo Summit Sno-Park sign and then the lodge for Adventure Mountain Tahoe, a winter sledding hill. Park in the parking lot, and then walk to its western edge where you will see a PCT and TRT sign. The trail parallels Highway 50 west through a mostly level to gently downhill lightly forested area with some large red fir, western white pine, and lodgepole pine. You meet a dirt road 0.7 mile from the start; cross the road, turn right, and then cross above a creek to adjacent Highway 50. Cross this very busy highway to where the trail resumes on the other side.

Now the trail heads uphill through a thicker forest for 0.2 mile to Johnson Pass Road, the access road that you would take if you were starting at Echo Lake. You cross the road, head up a steep embankment, and see a swift-moving stream to the left. With 1.1 miles to go to Lower Echo Lake, the trail crosses the stream, which could be challenging when it is filled with midsummer snowmelt. Walk through a lush and moist forest that will hold the snow until midsummer and then provide late summer wildflowers. Soon after, you pass several summer cabins and head downhill to the Lower Echo Lake's parking area. Cross this large paved parking lot and another smaller dirt parking lot to a short trail. You will find restroom facilities and the Echo Lakes Chalet Store here before you cross the lake's dam and reach the main trailhead.

Getting There from Lower Echo Lake From South Lake Tahoe drive west on Highway 50 to Echo Summit. From Echo Summit, drive 1 mile and turn right on Johnson Pass Road. Take this road 0.6 mile to a junction, where you will turn left on Echo Lakes Road. Go an additional 0.9 mile to a large parking lot above the lake. The resort requests that people using the trail not park in

Dicks Pass above Dicks Lake

the lower parking lot near the lake. You reach the trail by walking from the Echo Lakes Chalet Store and the lower parking lot over the dam to a TRT sign. This section of the TRT is also part of the Tahoe-Yosemite Trail and the Pacific Crest Trail. It is one of the more popular trails into Desolation Wilderness.

Getting There, Barker Pass to Echo Lake and Summit Take Highway 89 (West Lake Blvd.) about 4.25 miles south from Tahoe City, and turn right onto Blackwood Canyon Road, starting opposite Kaspian Beach. Drive 7 miles to the crest above Blackwood Canyon to where the paved road turns to dirt, and then continue another 0.2 mile to the PCT Trailhead dirt parking lot on your right. To access the trail, walk south across the dirt road and uphill about 50 yards.

Barker Pass Road is closed during the winter months. The road has a gate at the entrance and another one 2.5 miles farther, just above where it crosses Blackwood Creek. The road is not plowed, and these gates stay closed until the snow is melted to the top of Barker Pass. If you are planning to use the Barker Pass

Trailhead before mid-July, contact the TRTA to make sure that the road is open. Drive carefully on this narrow road since it is popular for bike riding and rollerblading.

Trail Description

From Lower Echo Lake's dam, the trail heads initially east and uphill, and near a switchback west you have a view toward South Lake Tahoe and Meyers. Especially prominent from the view is the effects of the 2007 Angora Fire, which came within a few miles (and a solid band of granite) of reaching Echo Lake. You walk west above the northern shore of long, narrow Lower Echo Lake. Your route is mostly minor ups and downs, bordered by spectacular granite formations, the deep blue lake, and mountains. The most dramatic granite cliff towering above you to the north is topped with a flagpole, which explains its name, Flagpole Peak (8363 feet).

The trail rambles for about 1 mile and passes a few gnarled junipers and Jeffrey pines that are hanging on through cracks in the granite. Then it ascends above lakeshore cabins. Your footing becomes more challenging as the terrain becomes rockier. You pass the west end of Lower Echo Lake. Magnificent views of the entire lake open up, and you will see some more charming rustic cabins along its granite shore. If you yell at Echo Lakes on a nice calm day, you are supposed to hear an echo.

After a traverse, you then curve south over the rocky peninsula between Lower and Upper Echo Lakes. At 2.5 miles you come to a junction. A left turn takes you on a short trail down to a pier, which provides access to Upper Echo Lake and the Echo Lakes Water Taxi. The taxi pier is also a great location for an afternoon swim.

Continue on the TRT from the junction, and climb steadily on more rocky terrain. You can enjoy breathtaking views of both Upper and Lower Echo Lakes from this section of trail. Upper Echo Lake is especially striking with its multiple granite islands topped with windblown trees. At 0.6 mile from the boat taxi, your trail levels off briefly, and you arrive at the boundary of Desolation Wilderness. Hiking beyond this point requires a permit, which you can get at the trailhead or through the Forest Service (permit information is found in Chapter 1, page 5). You will be hiking in Desolation Wilderness for more than 20 miles on the Tahoe Rim Trail. Just past the wilderness boundary you reach a junction. To your right, there is a trail that leads steeply uphill to Triangle Lake, with access to Echo Peak (8895 feet) (see side trip "Triangle Lake").

SIDE TRIP Triangle Lake

The side trail near the Desolation Wilderness boundary leads first to Triangle Lake and then over a steep ridge down to just east of Lily Lake and then by road down to Fallen Leaf Lake. The steep downhill trip is pretty with many lush stream crossings loaded with early summer wildflowers. The trail faces north, however, with snow lasting well into the summer. If you hike this section before July you may find several dangerous icy spots.

You continue on the TRT and PCT, climbing 0.5 mile to a junction on your left that leads to nearby Tamarack Lake. The trail to this charming lake is located 3.6 miles from the Echo Lakes Trailhead (and just 1.1 miles from the taxi), just inside the wilderness boundary. While it is a great place to stop, its proximity to the trailhead means it is usually very busy. Your views are glorious with imposing Ralston Peak (9235 feet) to the south and Echo Peak to the northeast.

After another 0.7 mile of rocky climbing, you reach another junction on your right, also leading toward Fallen Leaf Lake. I've hiked this section dozens of time, and each time I stumble along in frustration over the rocky and tricky footing. Am I the only one who fantasizes about several hundred sledgehammers pounding these rocks into submission? The climb west finally abates in 0.4 mile at a junction in Haypress Meadows. Here you encounter a mixed forest of red firs, mountain hemlocks, and western white pines scattered around small grassy meadows that bloom with wildflowers throughout the spring and summer, and perhaps most importantly, a smooth walking tread. The trail southwest

Susie Lake and the Crystal Range

heads over to Lake of the Woods, as does a southbound one 300 yards later. About 150 yards past it you meet a trail descending north to lovely Lake Lucille and Lake Margery.

About 0.3 mile later, at 5.2 miles from your trailhead, you meet another junction. The left turn takes you 0.5 mile west down to the southeast corner of Lake Aloha (from where you can wind 0.75 mile west over to the lake's 20-foot-high dam just above granite-lined America Lake). The TRT and PCT go straight ahead, through an area thick with midsummer wild-flowers, to the east shore of Lake Aloha in 0.8 mile. This heav-ily forested trail section may be covered in snow through early summer.

Lake Aloha (8116 feet) provides an incredible, unique land-scape. There are only a few wind-beaten trees surrounding the lake, but hundreds of small flat rock islands are scattered across its surface. The Crystal Range, a huge ridge of granite, topped by pointy Pyramid Peak (9983 feet) in the south, and Mt. Price (9976 feet) in the north, rises right up from the western shores of the lake. The trail meanders between granite boulders hugging the shore of Lake Aloha. Above the lake to the east is Cracked Crag, a big pile of rocks that families of marmots call home.

Heather Lake and the Crystal Range

Along the entire length of the barren landscape above Lake Aloha, you will find great swimming and camping spots. Aloha is one of my favorite places to take children camping. The little islands are fun to swim to, and the expanses of flat granite are perfect to stretch out on and gaze at Pyramid Peak. A dam controls the waters of Lake Aloha, and the lake shrinks dramatically in the fall. That great waterside spot you visited in June may be a long distance from the shore after Labor Day. In fact, the watermasters can let the water out of the lake very quickly. I have seen the lake full, and then two weeks later and five feet lower, you could hardly recognize the place.

When you reach the northeast corner of the lake, you meet a junction, 1.4 miles from the last one. Straight ahead a trail goes over Mosquito Pass. (Sounds enticing doesn't it? It's actually quite nice and leads to lots of great lakes and camping spots.) The TRT turns right, following the sign, which reads GLEN ALPINE. With Freel Peak (10,881 feet) visible in the distance, the trail begins a descent, that in 0.5 mile will bring you to the north shore of Heather Lake. Along the way, you will pass stunning multicolored rocky panoramas, lots of flowing water, early summer wildflowers, hemlock, and mountain heather topped with its small red flowers. In early summer much of this area may be under snow. Heather Lake is a picturesque large mountain lake with several tree-topped islands. There are limited campsites above the lake. Your 0.3-mile traverse along the north side of the lake toward its outlet provides a special photo opportunity looking west: Heather Lake's biggest island is in the foreground, and the Crystal Range looms above the lake in the background.

Just past Heather Lake, a very unique phenomenon is often visible in spring or early summer. Where the outlet creek melts under the snow, it forms a snow tunnel. I have seen it when the entrance to the snowcave was 10 feet high and at least 30 feet deep. Stepping into the cave provides you with a shower as well as the sight of the sun filtering through the blue geodesic shapes of the suncups above.

You now walk over a low, rocky saddle and begin a short descent to Susie Lake, another beautiful Sierra lake, this one bordered by red rock and dotted with islands. Susie Lake is loaded with campsites near its shore, many of which are illegal. Camps are required to be at least 100 feet from the shores of any lake, and you may be cited if you camp any closer to the water. Unfortunately, Susie Lake can be quite busy because it is only about 4 miles from the popular Glen Alpine Trailhead above Fallen Leaf Lake. The trail circles about half of the lake and offers views of the very imposing Dicks Peak (9974 feet) to the northwest, Jacks Peak (9856 feet) to the west, and the saddle of Dicks Pass (north) 1600 feet above you. This awesome view may lose some of its appeal when you realize that Dicks Pass is your next major goal.

Consider stopping at Susie Lake to relax and swim before making the big jaunt up the hill (and Susie can be quite warm by midsummer). About halfway along your trip around the lake, just before you reach the outlet for Susie Lake, about 1 mile past Heather Lake's outlet and a little more than 9 miles from your trailhead, go around the bend to the right, and traverse the side of the hill about 50 yards to a tremendous viewpoint of Grass

Lake and Keiths Dome to the southeast. Then, return to the trail, and cross the outlet creek. In the spring this crossing can be quite a challenge. If the main crossing is too deep, try going slightly upstream to cross on the logs. Be careful whatever you choose. Across the creek (hopefully you are still dry), continue around Susie Lake on the rocky terrain. After 0.25 mile, the trail veers east away from the lake and heads downhill (yes downhill, all of which and more must be made up a little farther on). In about 0.5 mile you reach a junction. A right turn heads 3.8 miles to the Glen Alpine Trailhead above Fallen Leaf Lake. You, however, will continue straight ahead on the TRT. After a short distance of 0.4 mile, you meet another junction that will take you to Half Moon Lake (see side trip "Half Moon Lake").

A right leads you to Fallen Leaf Lake in 3.6 miles. From here, the TRT begins a climb of 3.5 miles to Dicks Pass at 9380 feet. After a steady uphill grind, climbing dozens of wide steps, you reach a junction at 0.6 mile from the Half Moon Lake trail junction. To visit Gilmore Lake, you can go an additional 0.2 mile straight ahead from the Dicks Pass and Gilmore Lake junction. Gilmore Lake is a large round lake bordered by big red firs and lodgepole pines that makes a pleasant spot for a visit or an overnight stay, especially if you want to hike up nearby Mt. Tallac (9735 feet), which is about 1.75 miles farther and about 1450 feet higher. Tallac's panoramic views of Lake Tahoe are considered among the best. At a little less than 11 miles from the Echo Lake Trailhead, Gilmore makes an excellent camping choice.

> **SIDE TRIP Half Moon Lake**
>
> Turning left at the junction just beyond the Glen Alpine Trailhead junction, you will be headed toward Half Moon Lake, which you will reach in just 1.2 miles. Alta Morris Lake is an additional 0.7 mile. These lakes are both worthwhile goals for another trip. They lie at the foot of Dicks Peak and Jacks Peak, at the edge of a massive cirque. They may be less crowded than lakes along the TRT and PCT.

Ahead the TRT is well graded. Starting gently, it then becomes a more moderate climb toward a conspicuous saddle. Along the

Half Moon Lake and Jacks Peak from the south side of Dicks Pass

way, the views of Susie Lake, Half Moon Lake, and Alta Morris Lake are magnificent. In the summer and sometimes as late as early fall, wildflowers grow in abundance here, especially paintbrush and lupine, which may be seen in huge fields of flowers. In the fall you may also see an occasional explorer's gentian. While much of the journey is treeless, you will pass several gnarled junipers, which have been battered by the wind, as well as hemlocks and western white pines.

The trail reaches the saddle between Dicks Pass and Dicks Peak. From this location, your north view includes all of Dicks Lake directly below, as well as Fontanillis Lake, Middle Velma Lake, and a wide panorama of mountains in the distance including Twin Peaks (8878 feet) about 20 miles away and on a clear day, Lassen Peak (10,457 feet) more than 130 miles away. Since the trail is covered in snow much of the year, it is important to understand the distinction between the saddle and the pass. While from the saddle it is another 200 feet of climbing to the pass, don't try to avoid the climb by starting toward Dicks Lake from the saddle. It is a very steep north-facing slope that is covered in

Lake Aloha

ice much of the year. To reach the pass, continue on the trail east past a few particularly twisted whitebark pines to a level, treeless pass at 9380 feet. You have now climbed 1100 feet over 2.9 miles, since the junction near Gilmore Lake.

Once you reach the top of the pass, you may be ready to collapse—I mean relax and enjoy the view. And what a view! To the south, you can see Lake Aloha, Pyramid Peak, and the tip of Mt. Price, Susie Lake, Half Moon Lake, Alta Morris Lake, and all the way south-southeast to Round Top (10,381 feet) about 20 miles away. Towering above you to the west is the very imposing Dicks Peak and, to the southeast, Jacks Peak, both bearing patches of snow throughout most of the year. The best viewpoint is actually just before the top of the pass on a flat rock to the south of the trail.

You've had your fun. Now 13.6 miles into your route, it is time for the long downhill to Dicks Lake. In the next 1.7 miles you drop about 900 feet via a number of switchbacks to a saddle above Dicks Lake. While the south-facing side of Dicks Pass is loaded with grasses and wildflowers growing in the volcanic soil and between the rocks, the north-facing side of fractured granite is dominated by thick stands of mountain hemlock with just a few grasses here and there. A north-facing slope near 9000 feet elevation on the western side of the Sierra holds a tremendous amount of snow for much of the year. Thus the growing season is too short for most trees except the hardy hemlock. In addition, the hemlock is so prolific that it shades out the competition. At the saddle east of and above Dicks Lake you meet a junction (see side trip "Emerald Bay").

A left at the saddle continues your TRT and PCT journey. After a 0.2-mile descent southeast, you reach a short spur trail south to Dicks Lake, a large lake with plenty of space along its shore to roam or camp. Tucked away on the shady north side of Dicks Peak, this lake may still be frozen over in July after a big winter. At about 15.5 miles from your trailhead, with about 17 easier miles to go, this locale may be a good one to spend the night. From the spur trail, your trail veers northwest and continues another 0.3 mile to Fontanillis Lake, one of my favorites. Exposed granite and a few scattered hardy trees surround Fontanillis Lake. The trail approaches the granite-lined lakeshore in about 0.3 mile, but it takes another 0.3 mile to reach its shore. You hike in and out of numerous little bays, all with glorious views of Dicks Peak hulking above. You pass many great lunch and swimming spots along the way (perhaps a bit cold for a swim, but how about a quick jump in?). At the end of the lake, at 0.3 mile farther, the trail crosses its outlet creek (another tough early season crossing) and descends toward Middle Velma Lake (see side trip "Upper Velma Lake," next page).

After crossing Fontanillis Lake's outlet creek, you begin a descent through a deep forest of mostly red firs. In 0.8 mile of

> **SIDE TRIP Emerald Bay**
>
> A right turn at the junction east and above Dicks Lake will take you to Emerald Bay in 4.9 miles via the Bay View Trail. Straight ahead, northwest, is a rock knob. With a quick scramble, you will discover tremendous views here. You can see Fontanillis Lake and Dicks Peak to the west and south, respectively.

SIDE TRIP **Upper Velma Lake**

For another interesting side trip, follow the creek you crossed as it falls down a steep granite slab almost 0.5 mile to Upper Velma Lake. The granite slab is steep enough that the water, which is usually quite shallow, cascades down the slope, but it is not steep enough to prevent you from walking right next to the water. A trail runs from Upper Velma Lake to Middle Velma Lake, where you can rejoin the Tahoe Rim Trail or head out to Emerald Bay. Or you can hike cross-country south from the bottom of the falls above Upper Velma Lake, up a drainage to a small unnamed lake tucked against the granite face. Here you meet the trail to Dicks Lake. A left turn here takes you out to Emerald Bay.

walking and about 400 feet of descent, you reach a junction where the TRT heads left (west). A right turn would lead you out to Emerald Bay, about 5 miles away. On the TRT in a short distance you see Middle Velma Lake, a large lake with many islands that makes a great camping or swimming spot, although like much of Desolation Wilderness, it can be quite popular in the summer. If you are continuing north, be aware that the next lake, Richardson Lake, is smaller and marshier. Its accessibility by 4-wheel-drive vehicles makes it less attractive to those backpackers hoping to enjoy a motor-free experience.

Once you have relaxed or camped at Middle Velma Lake, 17.5 miles from the Echo Lakes Trailhead, you continue your journey north along the TRT and PCT. This second half of the hike from the Velma Lakes to Barker Pass is dramatically different from the first half that began at Echo Lake. While the first half goes through the heart of Desolation Wilderness, with more rocks than trees and beautiful rock-lined lakes (and lots of people), you are now embarking on a 15-mile journey through forest with only one lake (and fewer people). Before you leave Middle Velma Lake, be sure to filter water: The next reliable source is Richardson Lake 8.3 miles north.

Shortly after you leave Middle Velma Lake, you meet a junction, 0.3 mile past the previous one. Here a trail heads west down to Camper Flat and provides access to a whole host of Desolation Wilderness lakes and the Rubicon River. From this intersection the TRT, PCT, and TYT turns north and in 0.3 mile crosses boggy lands bordering Middle Velma Lake's outlet creek. It then goes 0.9 mile gently uphill to a junction with the Phipps Pass Trail, which turns off to the right (see side trip "Meeks Bay").

The TRT and PCT continues for the next 4.4 miles after the junction with the Phipps Pass Trail to a junction with a faint trail, which heads over to Lake Genevieve. (This little-used trail is overgrown in many spots and is not recommended.) There are two important features along this 4.4-mile stretch. The first is seasonal Phipps Creek, reached after a 1.5-mile, mostly gentle descent. You could camp near it (if you must). The second is after a 2-mile, erratic ascent to a high point with a short spur trail west, from which you can survey the Rubicon River lands. Past this you descend 0.9 mile to the next trail junction. You pass several small meadows blooming with asters, Queen Anne's lace, groundsel, corn lilies, and elephant heads. Thru-hikers are the primary users of this lightly used section of trail. If you meet someone who is hiking all the way from Mexico to Canada, be sure to take advantage of the opportunity and talk to them about their experiences. They have already walked more than 1,100 miles and surely have some fascinating stories to tell. One thing is certain; if they have made it this far, they are persistent.

Beyond the junction with the trail to Lake Genevieve, the combined PCT and TRT begins by going downhill. You can enjoy the views of Mt. Tallac and Dicks Peak in the distance to the south. As the trail moves into a more densely forested area, you will be leaving Desolation Wilderness at its north boundary, about 1.5 miles past the junction. Then 0.75 mile north of the wilderness, traversing the base of Lost Corner

> **SIDE TRIP Meeks Bay**
>
> At this point, the Tahoe-Yosemite Trail parts company with the PCT and TRT. The Phipps Pass Trail heads about 12 miles to Meeks Bay (and the terminus of the TYT). Along the way, you pass Phipps Pass and Peak (9234 feet) and Rubicon, Stony Ridge, Shadow, and Crag Lakes, and Lake Genevieve. If you have been hiking all the way from Yosemite, you are almost home. A wonderful point-to-point hike starts at Emerald Bay and ends at Meeks Bay via the Velma Lakes and Phipps Pass. This 18-mile route takes you by a string of lakes and exceptional viewpoints.

Hikers cool their feet in Lake Aloha.

Mountain, you reach a minor saddle. Next, you head 0.7 mile down to the northwest corner of tree-lined Richardson Lake. This pleasant little lake has several nice campsites set among the trees, but look out for mosquitoes in the spring. Richardson Lake, about 6.7 miles from the Barker Pass Trailhead, is accessible via a 4-wheel-drive dirt road, so be prepared for outdoor recreational vehicles, the main users of the north shore campsites.

From Richardson Lake, the trail heads north, first descending the lower east slopes of Sourdough Hill and then proceeding west above Miller Meadows, beyond which it crosses two dirt roads. Just past the first road (about 2 miles from Richardson Lake) you cross Miller Creek, a good source of water and a potentially difficult creek to cross in the spring. The second road crossing, about 200 yards farther, is the very popular McKinney Rubicon OHV Trail, which heads east down to the McKinney Estates subdivision on the west shore of Lake Tahoe or west on a famously difficult stretch of 4-wheel-drive terrain to the Rubicon River.

Onward, your journey is pleasant as you pass through thick fir forest and occasional small meadows opulent with wildflow-

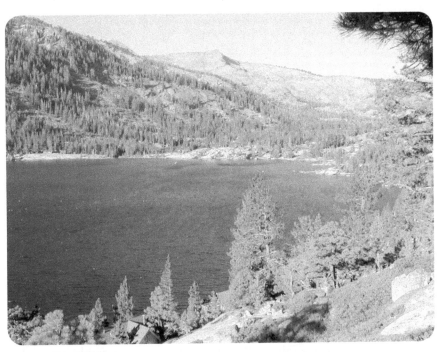

Lower Echo Lake

ers. The gently rolling terrain heads northwest 1.5 miles to Bear Lake's sparkling outlet creek and then 0.4 mile farther up to the Bear Lake Road.

Turn left on the road, walk about 50 yards to trail, and stay just above the road. You now have a 2-mile, 420-foot ascent to Forest Route 3. On it you will first pass one good-sized stream and then several smaller ones. Most of these streams host wildflowers until late summer. The trail climbs through Barker Meadows with several open slopes dotted with mules ears and views of Barker Peak, as well as the first sunshine in many miles of deep forest. Eventually you reach Barker Pass where the trail ends on a major dirt road, which provides access through Blackwood Canyon to Lake Tahoe. The PCT and TRT from Barker Pass to Tahoe City begins across the road and slightly to the west.

Barker Pass to Tahoe City

(16.7 miles)

Difficulty This moderate to strenuous section has several hefty climbs, but more of the trail runs downhill than uphill. The starting elevation is 7650 feet, and it ends near the Truckee River at about 6300 feet. If you are starting from the Tahoe City end, it is more strenuous.

Best Seasons This section can usually be hiked from late July to mid-October (or until the first major snowfall). Most of the first 7 miles of this section are at high elevations that receive a lot of snow. Much of the trail faces north or east—a combination that leads to a late snowmelt.

Highlights This section has beautiful ridgeline views of Lake Tahoe, Granite Chief Wilderness, both Blackwood and Ward Canyons, and lush areas loaded with wildflowers in both canyons. Twin Peaks (8878 feet), a Sierra Crest landmark, is accessible from the trail. In addition, there are numerous small stream crossings and several good camping spots. A lovely little waterfall cascades near one part of the trail in upper Ward Canyon. There is a pretty series of meadows known as Page Meadows. A dense forest area with huge pines and firs grows in the Ward Creek watershed. Wildlife is abundant and includes bear, coyote, raccoon, blue grouse, and perhaps goshawk and spotted owls.

Between Barker Pass and Twin Peaks this lakeless stretch tends to get less use than the trails in the Desolation Wilderness area, which has mountain lakes. However, in the Page Meadows vicinity, bikers, hikers, and joggers abound. At the end of your trip you may find that the Truckee River is a perfect place to swim or to complete your day with a rafting trip.

Page Meadows in the fall

Heads Up! In the fall, as streams dry up, the water supply can be limited. You reach the North Fork of Blackwood Creek, about 2.5 miles north of Barker Pass at the bottom of a meadow. In the next mile, you may find one or more springs before late summer. However, the most dependable water source is Ward Creek, about 8.5 miles north of Barker Pass. You parallel the creek, sometimes at a distance, for more than 3 miles, and by the time you're starting north from the canyon's main road you have only 5 miles to the Tahoe City Trailhead.

The only places to swim are the Truckee River at your destination and at adjacent Lake Tahoe. The Commons public beach is about 0.25 mile east of the TRT on Highway 28 in the center of Tahoe City. There are lots of junctions and turnoffs on this section of trail, and the Forest Service has been closing and rebuilding roads and trails in this area; follow the TRT trail markers, and pay attention to where you are going.

Barker Pass Road is not plowed and remains closed to cars until the snow melts in the spring or early summer. Often the road is not open until late June. The road is narrow in spots and is a favorite for bike riding. If you're a cyclist, observe the 20 mile-per-hour speed limit and watch for rollerbladers, rollerskiers, wayward dogs, and moms with strollers.

Tips for Mountain Bikers The first 5 miles of the TRT overlap with the PCT, and bikes are *not* allowed on the PCT. From Twin Peaks to Tahoe City, however, bikes are allowed: Start at 64 Acres in Tahoe City (also known as the Truckee River Access parking lot), follow the TRT along the Truckee River, and then head uphill rather steeply. In some places there are lots of loose rocks. After 1.7 miles, you reach the east edge of the Page Meadows area and a whole network of great biking trails. The TRT turns right at the first major junction (to the left, a trail crosses a small meadow and heads uphill into the trees) and provides a great gentle uphill ride through the forest above the perimeter of the meadows. In another 1.3 miles, you reach another junction, where you have two riding options.

Your first option: Turn left and follow the TRT as it skirts the edge of a meadow and crosses another one. The section of trail is built-up six inches above the meadow to protect the fragile ecosystem. After passing Page Meadows, the trail heads into the woods. At first the TRT follows a moderate downhill course, and then it descends more steeply on an old dirt road. Just 0.25 mile before reaching Ward Creek Blvd., the TRT turns right, becomes a single-track trail, and heads southwest. From here you go more gently downhill, a short distance to Ward Creek Blvd., a paved road leading to the Alpine Peaks subdivision. The TRT continues directly across the road.

Your second option: The alternative route to Ward Creek Boulevard and the TRT is to continue ahead for about 1 mile to the next major junction. Turn left and enjoy a fun downhill to Chamonix Road, a paved street in Alpine Peaks. Take Chamonix downhill to Courchevel, turn left, and head downhill. In a little more than 1 mile, you will see the TRT on your right. (Along the way the road name changes from Courchevel to Ward Creek Boulevard.)

From Ward Creek Blvd., the TRT follows an old dirt road for about 2 miles to a washed-out bridge. After the bridge, the trail starts uphill in earnest through a beautiful area of small meadows where aspens are interspersed with forests of tall old-growth trees. As the trail gets steeper, most bikers will walk their bikes or stop and turn around. Eventually, about 5.2 miles beyond Ward Creek Boulevard you reach a saddle between Twin Peaks on your right and Stanford Rock on the left. The trail to the right leads steeply uphill to Twin Peaks where bikes are *not* allowed. The trail to the left leads uphill very steeply to a great lookout point and then a 4-mile fun downhill on a dirt road to Ward Creek Boulevard. Just before reaching the road, you cross Ward Creek in an area that can be deep and difficult to ford until late summer.

The 4-mile section between Stanford Rock and Ward Creek is also challenging going the opposite direction as an uphill ride. The start is about 0.5 mile east of the TRT on Ward Creek Road. You will see a gated trail leading off from the road next to a large open flat area on the south side of the highway. Immediately after passing the gate you cross Ward Creek. The climb varies between moderately steep to very steep and provides tremendous views of the lake and Blackwood Canyon. Eventually you reach the Stanford Rock viewpoint and a spectacular view of Ward Canyon, Twin Peaks, and the Sierra Crest. After enjoying the view, turn left and follow the trail downhill to a junction with the TRT. Or you can turn around and ride back the way you came. If you choose to ride from here on the TRT, be prepared for a challenging and steep ride on loose soil, with several technical rocky sections.

Getting There, Barker Pass to Tahoe City Take Highway 89 (West Lake Blvd.) about 4.25 miles south of Tahoe City, and turn right onto Blackwood Canyon Road, starting opposite Kaspian Beach. Drive 7 miles to the crest above Blackwood Canyon to where the paved road turns to dirt and then another 0.2 mile to the dirt PCT Trailhead parking lot on your right.

Twin Peaks from the head of Ward Canyon

Getting There, Tahoe City to Barker Pass From the intersection of Highways 89 and 28 at the stoplight in Tahoe City, head south on Highway 89 about 0.25 mile to the Truckee River Access parking area (64 Acres). Park in the lot. The trail starts along the south side of the Truckee River. As you follow the Truckee River west and downstream, the trail begins as a bike trail. Continue to follow the river downstream as the bike trail leads into a paved road that then becomes a dirt road. Walk on the dirt road for 0.3 mile, and meet a gate right next to the Truckee River. Go around the gate and across a south-climbing gravel road to the start of the Tahoe Rim Trail.

Trail Description

At Barker Pass (7650 feet) the trail begins by traversing west around the south side of Barker Peak (8166 feet), where you get excellent views of Desolation Wilderness to the south. In 0.9 mile your moderately steep walk through a field of mules ears reaches the Sierra Crest, where you have views east down the expanse of Blackwood Canyon to Lake Tahoe. Beyond the crest, your route continues with a gentle ascent northeast across the canyon's upper

Volcanic plugs north of Barker Pass

slopes. In 0.25 mile you pass a beautiful stream bordered with aster, delphinium, tiger lily, columbine, and paintbrush, among other wildflowers.

After a pleasant walk gently up through mostly open volcanic terrain that is interrupted by a red fir forest, you cross a steep face to the base of two lofty volcanic plugs, about 0.5 mile past the stream. From here you have wide open views of Lake Tahoe and Blackwood Canyon to the east. From these lofty twin rock formations, the trail descends into a large bowl lush with wildflowers and greenery late into the summer. Mountain hemlock is now the dominant tree. These fascinating trees are laden with cones on their thick green foliage. The hemlock can be most easily identified by its drooping top, which gives it a fairy-tale appearance.

As you descend farther into this lovely bowl, you pass several areas graced by Sierra wildflowers including explorer's gentian, which blooms into the fall. At the bottom of the bowl, about 2.5 miles from the trailhead, is a great camping spot. It has a running stream (North Fork of Blackwood Creek), a nice flat place to rest your head, and views of Lake Tahoe and Blackwood Canyon. Just beyond this camping spot, the trail rounds a corner and continues to descend past several spring-fed creeks. It's a wildflower haven with late season water and a continuing series of views.

After about a 1-mile traverse from the camping spot, your trail starts a series of long switchbacks almost to the crest of the ridge. The climb begins in a dark viewless forest of large red fir trees. As you climb, you will see Ellis Peak to the southeast, Desolation Wilderness to the south, and almost all of Blackwood Canyon to the east. Just below the top of the crest, you round the ridge to find new views of the south side of Twin Peaks (8878 feet).

Then you pass the Granite Chief Wilderness sign and quickly reach the Sierra Crest, where there are views in all directions. To your north and west, you can see the full expanse of Granite Chief Wilderness, to the northeast, you see nearby Twin Peaks, to the east Lake Tahoe, and to the south Desolation Wilderness lies in the distance. In the foreground you can review the knife-edge ridge whose backside you just climbed.

Just 0.25 mile beyond this exposed viewpoint you meet a junction, at 4.8 miles from Barker Pass. This is where the TRT and PCT part ways after running together for a total of about 50 miles. Straight ahead are the PCT and Canada. A right turn takes you along the southern slope of Twin Peaks on the TRT. Those of you without the time or inclination to hike to Canada should turn right.

In 0.5 mile you meet a spur trail to the top of the eastern Twin Peak. (For those hiking south, this junction is about 6.2 miles from the Ward Canyon Trailhead.) If you are going to take this trail, be forewarned that it can be a bit treacherous, but the views are spectacular.

From the summit trail junction, continue descending along a ridgeline on the TRT for 1 mile through a mixed forest of red fir, hemlock, and western white pine to a saddle. Along the route you have scenic views of Squaw Valley and Alpine Meadows to the north. The saddle has nice dry campsites with views and

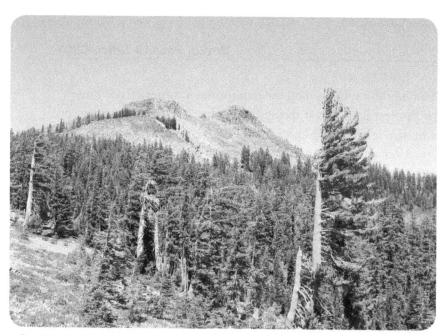
Twin Peaks and windswept trees

another junction. The TRT turns left, while the trail straight ahead continues to Stanford Rock, as described above in the mountain biking tips.

You are now heading north down a rather steep hill through a deep forest of fir and hemlock trees into Ward Canyon. This portion of the trail is bone-jarringly steep with loose dark soil, but the views, especially of Twin Peaks to your left, are glorious. After about 1.1 miles of downhill, you encounter a large meadow at the base of Twin Peaks. This beautiful meadow, surrounded by imposing peaks high above, is a splendid resting spot. Next, the descent is less steep and takes you into a more thinly forested section. You pass another meadow and then see 30-foot McCloud Falls, just off the trail on your left. Switchback down toward Ward Creek for 0.9 mile, and then pass several lush meadows that are surrounded by aspen trees, as well as large red firs and Jeffrey pines.

Cross Ward Creek on a wide bridge. The usually swiftly moving creek is a great place to take a break and soak your feet in the water before a few more dusty miles. Across the bridge you walk on a former road, which first traverses 0.5 mile and then heads gently downhill. After passing a washed-out bridge across a tributary of Ward Creek the trail joins an old dirt road. You can camp immediately past the bridge site, north of the road, in an opening in the trees, which the Forest Service used as a camp when they were building the TRT between here and Twin Peaks. You can usually find water in the creek or in a spring on the northeast edge of the camp.

The TRT heads gently downslope for 1.75 miles through meadows and forest on old roadbed to a trailhead on Ward Creek Boulevard, a paved road leading up to Alpine Peaks, a development on the "backside" (south) of Alpine Meadows Ski Area. Along this stretch of trail, there are several nice views, including one of Grouse Rock, which you can see from a particularly pretty meadow that borders Ward Creek on your right. (Grouse Rock is the large volcanic rock on the ridgeline to the west between Twin Peaks and Ward Peak that sits right above the Pacific Crest Trail. It is a popular destination with backcountry skiers.) You are following Ward Creek, but it is mostly unseen until you approach Ward Creek Blvd. Your trail, blocked at the trailhead by a gate, was once used regularly as an off-highway vehicle route. In the New Year's floods of 1997, the road was washed-out in several locations. Where it was once smooth dirt, the trail in many places became a jumble of rocks after the soil washed away.

At Ward Creek Boulevard you see a TRT kiosk. With 5 miles to go to Tahoe City, cross the road and begin climbing through a forest of white fir and Jeffrey pine. After about 0.25 mile the trail turns left onto a dirt road and heads uphill more steeply. Near the top of the hill, Ward Canyon, Ward Peak, and the Sherwood chairlift at Alpine Meadows Ski Area are visible through an opening in the trees.

After a steep 0.6 mile, the trail levels at a junction with another dirt road. A right turn here would take you to eastern Page Meadows and the Talmont Estates development in about 1 mile. The TRT angles left and winds up through a young forest for 0.4 mile to the road's end, where posts were installed to block vehicles. Here a lateral trail heads left to the lowest of the Page Meadows

SIDE TRIP **Oven**

Just off this lateral trail is an oven built by Basque sheepherders. Built in the 1950s, the oven provides evidence of a unique lifestyle once present in Page Meadows. Sit next to the oven, and imagine sheepherders enjoying freshly baked bread while watching sheep graze in the meadow under the beautiful aspen trees. If you continue on the lateral trail through the meadow leading to Alpine Peaks, you will find lots of flowers, aspens, and a clear-running stream.

and provides access to the Alpine Peaks neighborhood about 0.25 mile away (see side trip "Oven").

You are now in the Page Meadows area, a series of five interconnected meadows that serve as a popular retreat for hiking, mountain biking, and cross-country skiing. The meadows provide an easily accessible outdoor haven for many residents who live in nearby developments. They are especially popular as a place to go cross-country skiing on full moon nights.

From the trail that headed to the oven, the TRT goes straight ahead through the road gate and follows the meadow area on your left for a short distance before entering a large meadow. The trail is built up 6 inches above the meadow to prevent damage to this fragile ecosystem. About a third of the way across this beautiful meadow, you meet a trail starting east. It provides access to three other large meadows, as well as a route to Tahoe City. The TRT continues straight. At the end of the meadow, turn around to enjoy a tree-framed view of Twin Peaks. Are you a yogi? This is a great place for a headstand. Your trail now heads north out of the meadow, into a grove of aspens before entering a forest of fir trees. About 0.2 mile from the meadow you meet another junction (see side trip "Alpine Meadows").

SIDE TRIP **Alpine Meadows**

At the junction north of the meadow with that good Twin Peaks view, a spur trail leads left (west). In about 3 miles you would reach the Alpine Meadows residential area. In addition, spurs from this trail lead to the top of Scott Peak, the Alpine Meadows Ski Area, or Tahoe City via the bike trail along the Truckee River. These trails are fun mountain biking routes or pleasant hikes through the forest.

The TRT turns right (east), however, and parallels the mostly unseen meadows on your right. The next 1.3 miles are primarily downhill, with several short uphills. This is a very popular mountain biking section for a good reason. It rolls along with lots of fun little twists and turns on a fairly smooth surface. The trail levels near the edge of a small meadow, and you meet another junction (see side trip "Rawhide Drive").

The TRT turns left (east) and begins a 0.6-mile steep descent down a narrow canyon, with rocky and challenging (for bikes) terrain, to a junction. The TRT veers left. If you are on your bike and would like to avoid this difficult section, refer to the side trip "Rawhide Drive" for an easier route to Tahoe City. From the TRT marker, you travel almost 1 mile, generally downhill, winding through the shade of the fir and sugar pine trees until you arrive at a trail junction on the Truckee River. Turn right and follow the trail 0.1 mile east to a gravel road where the trail tread ends. You now walk across the road and past a gate. Stop here to swim in the Truckee River or to watch summer rafters. Your trail is now a dirt road heading along the river

> **SIDE TRIP   Rawhide Drive**
>
> A right turn at the junction in the small meadow leads across a snippet of meadow, and then after a short uphill, it runs into a major trail. A right-hand turn on this trail junction will take you to the biggest meadow in the Page Meadows area in 0.5 mile. Turn left at the trail junction and in 1.5 miles downhill, you reach Rawhide Drive, close to Tahoe City. If you want to head toward Tahoe City at this point, follow Rawhide north to Granlibakken Road, turn right, and follow Granlibakken Road to West Lake Boulevard, also known as Highway 89. Turn left on the bike trail, and in 0.5 mile you will be in Tahoe City.

upstream 0.3 mile to a paved road. The National Forest 64 Acres (Truckee River Access) parking lot is straight ahead.

From the parking lot, a 0.3-mile walk along bike paths and roads reaches the beginning of the next section of the TRT, from Tahoe City to Brockway Summit (Section 1, page 71). Follow the bike trail to the pedestrian bridge across the Truckee River to Highway 89. Turn right, and follow the bike trail 50 yards to its end. Cross Highway 89 to Fairway Drive, which is directly across the highway. Go 0.2 mile up Fairway Drive to the Fairway Community Center parking lot on your right. The TRT continues across the street.

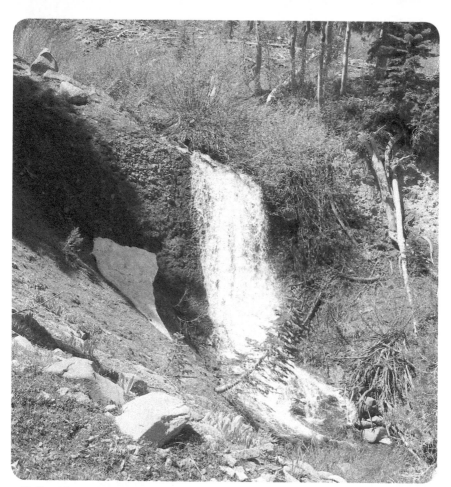

McCloud Falls in Ward Canyon

Other Tahoe Area Attractions and Activities

Once you have exhausted all of the recreation possibilities on the Tahoe Rim Trail, you may want to check out some other Tahoe area trails. Here are brief summaries of a few of my favorites.

Hiking

Emerald Bay

Difficulty Easy. Depending on where you go, it is anywhere from 2 to 9 miles.

Map *Tahoe Rim Trail Map 2, Section 7*

Best Seasons Do this hike in early spring or later in the fall. After a mild winter, you can hike it from April through December.

Highlights Emerald Bay provides many great hiking opportunities. On the edge of a beautiful sandy beach at the western edge of the bay is the Vikingsholm Castle with its granite touches, carved wood spikes and gargoyles, roof covered with wildflowers, and its gorgeous stained-glass windows. The castle was constructed from 1928 to 1929 by Mrs. Lora Knight, after she had purchased 239 acres at the end of Emerald Bay for $250,000. Trails lead from the Vikingsholm to a beautiful waterfall and along both sides of Emerald Bay.

Heads Up! During the summer, these trails (especially the 1-mile portion from the parking lot to the Vikingsholm) can be very busy! The best time to go is on a weekday in early spring or late fall when you will be more likely to have the place to yourself.

Getting There From Tahoe City, drive 17 miles south on Highway 89 to the Vikingsholm parking lot located on the south side of the road (10 miles north of the intersection of Highways 50 and 89 in South Lake Tahoe). During the summer, this lot can be full early in the day. An alternative parking area is located a quarter mile farther south on Highway 89 at the Eagle Falls Trailhead. There is a fee to use either lot.

Brief Trail Description The trail from the parking lot to the Vikingsholm is a gentle descent for a mile. Two trails lead out from the Vikingsholm. The first takes you 1.5 miles along the north side of Emerald Bay, in and out of sandy inlets, past the Emerald Bay Boat Campground, and to Emerald Point. This south-facing section of trail is the first area to emerge from the winter snows. From Emerald Point, the trail continues across a small peninsula and heads north for 3 miles along the lakeshore to Bliss State Park (along the way keep your eyes open for ospreys and eagles).

A second trail leaves the Vikingsholm and heads southwest a short distance to a junction at a bridge across Eagle Creek. A right turn leads you up to Eagle Falls in a third of a mile. The falls are quite dramatic when they are filled with springtime runoff. If you turn left, you will cross Eagle Creek, travel past the Emerald Bay landslide of 1955, then continue along the southern side of the bay to Emerald Bay Campground, 1.5 miles from Vikingsholm.

Loch Leven Lakes

Difficulty It is a moderately difficult, but well-graded climb to the first of the three Loch Leven Lakes. The journey between the lakes is an easy ascent. If you visit all the lakes and return, it is a total distance of a little less than 8 miles.

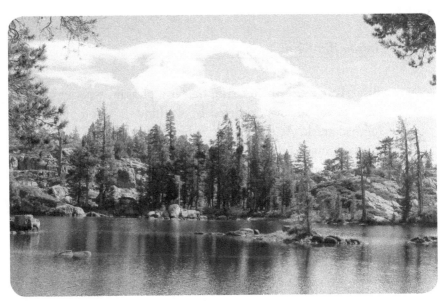
Loch Leven Lakes

Best Seasons Late June to late October. The trail is at a relatively low elevation (5880 feet), but it faces north in an area that receives much snow.

Highlights This hike is 30 miles closer to the Bay Area and Sacramento than most other Sierra hikes. It is also easily accessible via Interstate 80. In just a few miles you can reach three wonderful lakes lying on granite benches. The two farthest lakes provide good camping opportunities and excellent swimming in relatively warm water. These lakes make especially attractive locations for family camping trips, since they are great to explore and easy enough for many families to reach.

Heads Up! This trail's easy accessibility keeps Loch Leven Lakes busy throughout the summer. You will almost certainly not have the lakes to yourself.

Getting There Take Interstate 80 to the Big Bend Exit, which is 1.5 miles east of Cisco Grove and 6 miles west of Soda Springs. Drive about 1 mile south on Hampshire Rocks Road (Old Highway 40), past the Rainbow Lodge, and park on the right at the trailhead parking lot. It has a pit toilet and parking space for about ten vehicles.

Brief Trail Description The trail is a pleasant woodsy walk up past several streams bordered by wildflowers before it crosses a railroad track. At that point, it begins a moderate, well-graded climb through a thick forest of firs and pines. In a little less than 3 miles from the trailhead, you reach Upper Loch Leven Lake, followed in 0.3 mile by Middle Loch Leven Lake, and then at 3.9 miles from the trailhead, my favorite of the three, High Loch Leven Lake. Also nearby is Salmon Lake, accessed via a trail near the lowest lake. It is also shallow and warm and is unique for the Tahoe Sierra in that it has catfish.

Winnemucca Lake and Round Top Lake

Difficulty Easy to moderately difficult. This is a fairly short hike, only 2.5 miles to Winnemucca Lake and 3.4 miles to Round Top Lake, with a round-trip distance of 6.8 miles. The high elevation of this trail may make it moderately difficult for hikers unaccustomed to high altitudes. The trail starts at 8590 feet with Round Top Lake sitting at 9350 feet. A faint trail also leads from Round Top Lake up a very steep mile to the summit of Round Top (10,381 feet). If you add Round Top to your itinerary, this hike is strenuous.

Best Seasons Late July through October. This hike is in a high-elevation area that receives a tremendous amount of snow, which can last till midsummer.

Highlights If you are looking for relatively easy access to some tremendous high mountain scenery, this is a great choice. The area between Carson Pass and Winnemucca Lake hosts an incredible variety of wildflowers from late July through August. The prolific flower display may include lupine, elephant head, gentian, delphinium, monkeyflower, tiger lily, columbine, rein orchid, and a full palette of paintbrushes. The area around Round Top Lake and the accompanying peak has a rugged appeal and is a popular destination for summertime skiers and snowboarders, who are trying to find that last patch of snow. This hike is a good choice for those in the South Lake Tahoe area, which is only about 25 miles away.

Heads Up! Permits are required to camp in the Mokelumne Wilderness Area, where much of this hike takes place. During the summer, permits are available at the trailhead at Carson Pass. During the rest of the year, you need to contact the Amador Ranger District in Jackson, California, at (209) 295-4251. Given the short distance to the lakes and the fragility of this high-altitude location, it is best to dayhike this trail.

Getting There The trail starts from Carson Pass near Kirkwood Ski Area south of Lake Tahoe. From Meyers, take Highway 89 south about 11 miles to the intersection of Highways 88 and 89 (Picketts Junction). Be sure to come to a complete stop at this remote intersection since the California Highway Patrol watches it closely. Turn right on Highway 88, and go approximately 9 miles through Hope Valley and up to Carson Pass. There is a parking area on your left just as the road reaches the summit. The trailhead also has an information center (in summers only).

Brief Trail Description From the Carson Pass parking lot, your route is a gentle-to-moderate ascent for 2.5 miles to Winnemucca Lake. You pass incredible summertime wildflower displays in the open areas below Winnemucca Lake. A mile more of moderate climbing brings you to Round Top Lake, which sits in a basin just below huge rocky crags and Round Top (10,381 feet). From here you can follow a faint very steep trail to the top of Round Top, where you will find 360-degree, awe-inspiring views. Your views to the north include Lake Tahoe and a number of high peaks surrounding it, including Freel Peak (10,881 feet), Mt. Tallac (9735 feet), Pyramid Peak (9983 feet), and on a clear day, Mt. Rose (10,776 feet), some 46 miles away. The last few hundred feet at the top of the mountain is steep, crumbly volcanic rock. Stop where the ridgetop trail meets the steep rock, for equally spectacular views without the added danger.

Crag Lake

Difficulty Easy to moderately difficult

Map *Tahoe Rim Trail Map 2, Section 7*

Best Seasons Mid-June to mid-October. This trail provides late spring access to eastern Desolation Wilderness.

Highlights Crag Lake is an especially magnificent spot with the high granite slab of Crag Peak looming over the lake. This hike is the easiest route into Desolation Wilderness from the Tahoe Basin, and it usually is snow-free a month earlier than Eagle Falls, Bay View, and Echo Lake, the other Tahoe area trailheads used to access Desolation Wilderness. Both lakes are great locations for swimming or camping.

Heads Up! This trail is quite popular for both dayhiking and camping, so parking can be limited in the summer. A permit is required to enter Desolation Wilderness. Dayhiking permits are available at the trailhead. For backpacking permits contact the Forest Service office in South Lake Tahoe at (530) 573-2694.

Getting There From Tahoe City, drive 10 miles south on Highway 89 to Meeks Bay (this is about 17 miles north of the intersection of Highways 50 and 89 at the South Lake Tahoe "Y"). The trailhead is on the west side of Highway 89 at the bend in the road.

Brief Trail Description This trail starts out as a level walk through widely scattered forest and a wildflower-dotted meadow and then heads up into the trees following the path of Meeks Creek. In 4.6 miles you reach Lake Genevieve and Crag Lake shortly thereafter. If you would like to hike farther, you can continue past Stony Ridge Lake and Rubicon Lake, before heading over Phipps Pass to the Tahoe Rim Trail and Middle Velma Lake. From Middle Velma Lake, Emerald Bay is only 5 miles away, making for a spectacular 18-mile point-to-point hike.

Crag Lake and Peak

Fontanillis and Velma Lakes Loop

Difficulty Strenuous, 12-mile loop with 2000 feet of elevation gain

Map *Tahoe Rim Trail Map 2, Section 7*

Best Seasons Mid-July to early October

Highlights Here is Desolation Wilderness in all its splendor, with spectacular views of granite peaks, mountain lakes, and a variety of plant life. Eagle, Granite, Fontanillis, and Dicks Lakes, as well as all three Velma Lakes, are excellent for swimming or camping.

Heads Up! These trails, especially on the first mile to Eagle Lake, can be crowded in the summer. Day use and backpacking permits are required. Day-use permits are available at the trailhead. To get a backpacking permit, contact the Forest Service office at (530) 573-2694.

Getting There You can start from either of two trailheads, both of which are located at the western end of Emerald Bay on Highway 89. The Eagle Lake and Eagle Falls Trailhead is about

200 yards south of the Vikingsholm parking lot, which is about 17 miles south of Tahoe City and 10 miles north of South Lake Tahoe. There is a fee for parking. The Bay View Campground and Trailhead is 1 mile south of the Eagle Falls Trailhead on Highway 89, across from the vista parking area. Drive through the campground to its western edge where you will find trailhead parking.

Brief Trail Description The Eagle Lake Trail ascends about 1 mile to often crowded Eagle Lake. Then you stay left and climb steadily and sometimes steeply along the slope of south Maggies Peak to a junction 2.6 miles from the trailhead. If you are starting from the Bay View Trailhead, you hike about 0.5 mile to a stunning view of Emerald Bay and then another half mile to Granite Lake. Next is a steep set of switchbacks into the cleavage between Maggies Peaks. These breast-shaped mountains, also known as Round Buttons, were named after Maggie. Who was she? Legend has it that she was a buxom barmaid at the Tahoe Tavern Resort.

The Bay View Trail reaches the saddle between the two peaks and then descends to a junction and a meeting with the Eagle Lake Trail. From here, with both trails as one, you hike along rolling rocky terrain for a little less than a mile to a junction, where you take a left turn onto the trail leading to Dicks Lake. Now in the heart of the stark Desolation Wilderness, land of granite boulders, sandy soils, and scattered trees, you go about 0.5 mile to a beautiful pond. This shallow body of water is a good swimming spot, and is especially pretty in the fall when the mountain heather surrounding the lake turns bright red. Your journey ascends across a granite slab to a saddle and junction. A left turn climbs up to Dicks Pass, but your right turn takes you to Dicks and Fontanillis Lakes. You are now on the Tahoe Rim Trail and Pacific Crest Trail. (For more detailed information on the next 2 miles of trail refer to the TRT description in Chapter 6, page 157). In 0.2 mile you meet another junction, with a left turn going to Dicks

Lake in 100 yards, and a right turn heading to Fontanillis, your next destination. At Dicks Lake, look for osprey diving for fish in the evening. The trail follows along Fontanillis Lake and finally reaches its outlet creek.

The trail crosses the creek and heads downhill for about a mile along a ridge to a junction. If you turn left, you will be heading to Middle Velma Lake on the PCT and TRT. However, you should turn right, leave the TRT and PCT, and head uphill for a little more than a mile back to the Dicks Lake junction, and then retrace your steps back to the Bay View and Eagle Falls Trails junction. Hopefully, you left a car at both trailheads, which will enable you to hike a loop back to Emerald Bay via a different trail than where you began.

Donner to Squaw Valley

Difficulty A strenuous hike of about 15 miles

Best Seasons Mid-July to mid-October. Patches of snow can last until August on the north-facing slope of Anderson Peak.

Highlights This section of the Pacific Crest Trail provides miles of stunning 360-degree views from atop a windswept ridge. Ridgecrest views reach all the way from Mt. Rose in the northeast, to Lake Tahoe, in the southeast, with the Granite Chief Wilderness to the south and west. You will see a wide variety of terrain and wildflower species, including large fields of mules ears. This well-constructed trail has firmly packed, sandy soils good for fast-moving, long-distance hikers or runners. Everyone will enjoy its high-altitude remoteness. When Desolation Wilderness is packed with people, you may only encounter a few people on this trail. The trail goes by Roller Pass, a portion of the original Emigrant Trail used by pioneers when they came to California.

Heads Up! Very little water is available on the trail, and if you are hiking in late summer or fall, assume that there will be no water. Early in the summer, a northeast-facing 100-foot-long section about 3 miles into the trail may be treacherous if it is still covered with snow. Most of the trail is treeless and exposed to the sun and wind; be sure to bring plenty of sunscreen and a windbreaker. Your trail intersects with a variety of use paths descending from Shirley Canyon along the last mile of your route. Take care to avoid getting lost.

Getting There Take Interstate 80 to the Soda Springs exit, and drive 4 miles east on Highway 40 to Donner Summit (Sugar Bowl Academy will be on your right). Take a right turn at the summit, just before the road starts to go downhill, and go 0.2 mile to the trailhead on your left. This point-to-point hike requires a shuttle; be sure to leave a vehicle behind Olympic Village Inn in Squaw Valley.

Brief Trail Description Climb south on the Pacific Crest Trail, where in 1 mile you reach a junction with the Mt. Judah Loop trail. This alternate route heads up to Mt. Judah, which has excellent views, and then circles back and meets the PCT, adding 0.4 mile to your hike's length. About 2 miles into the hike you reach a saddle, Roller Pass. Just off the trail to the southeast, the Donner Party of 1846 winched their wagons up the steep slope below. Another 0.3 mile of gentle climbing brings you to another saddle below Mt. Lincoln. From here, the trail traverses a steep slope and then follows the ridgecrest with views in all directions for several miles to Anderson Peak. Your trail circles Anderson Peak and then climbs another ridge for a 1-mile journey to Tinker Knob, where a short use trail takes you to its summit.

At 8 miles into your hike, the trail descends from Tinker Knob into a deep wide bowl (North Fork of American River Canyon) with wildflowers and sparse tree cover. You cross this bowl and then begin a steady climb, and at 4 miles from Tinker Knob, you reach a junction. Head east (left) on a steady downhill for 3 miles into Squaw Valley.

Aloha Lake Loop via Tamarack Trail

Difficulty This 12-mile loop is strenuous overall. The first 2.5 miles are very strenuous.

Map *Tahoe Rim Trail Map 1, Section 7*

Best Seasons Mid-July through Mid-October

Highlights This is a classic hike into the heart of Desolation Wilderness with views of more than a dozen lakes, numerous high granite and volcanic peaks, and a tremendous variety of mountain terrain.

Heads Up! The first few miles up a canyon to a saddle are very steep, with almost 2000 feet of elevation gain. While not mountain climbing, it is certainly one of the steepest sections of trail I have ever hiked. It is especially difficult if you are carrying a heavy backpack. In the early summer this steep section can be icy and requires extra caution.

Getting There Go about 0.5 mile west of Camp Richardson on Highway 89, and turn south on Fallen Leaf Lake Road (about 3 miles northwest of the intersection of Highways 50 and 89 in South Lake Tahoe). Follow this road 5.3 miles along the edge of Fallen Leaf Lake to the Glen Alpine Trailhead. The first 4.5 miles of the route are one and one-half lanes wide, and the last 0.8 mile is only one lane wide. From the Glen Alpine parking area, walk on Fallen Leaf Lake Road back toward the lake about 0.25 mile to the Tamarack Trail on the right-hand (south) side.

Brief Trail Description Hike 2.5 steep miles to a level junction with the Triangle Lake Trail. These first few miles are extremely beautiful. You will hike through lush, almost junglelike stream crossings with tiger lilies and columbines and then climb through open areas of granite boulders from which you can enjoy great views. From the Triangle Lake junction, go straight and climb more gently now to an open, almost treeless, viewpoint that faces

Echo Lakes and Ralston Peak. Then, proceed downhill to a junction where the Tahoe Rim Trail and Pacific Crest Trail climbs up from Echo Lakes. Turn right on the PCT and TRT, and follow the signs to Lake Aloha. For a more detailed description of the next 6 miles of trail along the TRT, refer to Section 7 (page 157).

When you reach Lake Aloha, turn right, and head north along Aloha's eastern shore to a junction at its northern edge, where you turn right. In the next 2 miles you descend past two beautiful lakes, Heather and Susie. From Susie Lake you hike about 0.5 mile to a junction where you turn right. Now leaving the PCT and TRT you hike 0.5 mile to another junction, turn right, and follow it 3.3 miles, mostly downhill, to the Glen Alpine Trailhead where your car is parked.

Mountain Biking

Page Meadows and Ward Canyon

Difficulty This area has a whole system of interconnected trails, which vary from easy to strenuous.

Map *Tahoe Rim Trail Map, Section 8*

Best Seasons Late June through late October. *Do not ride through the meadows when they are wet.*

Highlights These trails have it all: rolling forested terrain, lush green meadows in the summer, and glorious yellow and red leaves in the fall. It is a fun, smooth single-track trail with good climbs and thrilling descents. The variety of trails encourages you to visit again and again.

Heads Up! The meadow areas are fragile when wet and should be avoided. Sometimes the elaborate trail network can be confusing. You may end up coming out somewhere different than you think you will, but that's part of the fun.

Getting There Five different locations access this great network of dirt roads and single-track trails.

1. **Granlibakken Road:** Go 0.5 mile south of Tahoe City on Highway 89, turn right on Granlibakken Road, and then turn left on Rawhide, which you take to its end. The trail starts behind a gate.

2. **End of Silvertip in Talmont Estates:** Take Highway 89 about 2 miles south of Tahoe City, and turn right on Pine Street. Then turn right on Tahoe Park Heights, right on Big Pine, and left on Silvertip, which you follow to its end.

3. **Ward Canyon Boulevard:** Go south from Tahoe City about 2.5 miles on Highway 89. Turn right on Pineland Drive. At the end of the straightaway, veer left and follow the WARD CANYON sign. Go about 1 mile to the TRT on your right side, and start climbing.

4. **Chamonix:** Follow the directions to #3 above, and go an additional mile on Ward Canyon Boulevard, which becomes Courchevel. Turn right on Chamonix, and go to the end of the road where a trail heads west.

5. **Snowcrest Road, Alpine Meadows:** Take Highway 89 about 3.5 miles north from Tahoe City to Alpine Meadows Road, where you turn left. Go about 1 mile, and turn left on Snowcrest. Follow this road to a gated dirt road on your left.

Brief Trail Description Since there are so many different entrances and a complicated network of trails, I do not give exact directions for this trip. A number of loop trails go around Page Meadows, up to the top of Scott Peak at Alpine Meadows, or into the Tahoe City and Rawhide area. One loop starts at Rawhide, goes over to Snowcrest, and then heads back along the bike trail between Alpine Meadows and Tahoe City. Another trail starts at

Mountain bikers on the East Shore

Chamonix, goes around the meadows, and then loops back to the same starting point or down to Ward Canyon Boulevard. Explore the area and see where you end up.

Tahoe Cross-Country Ski Area and Burton Creek State Park

Difficulty Moderate. A variety of trails and loops provide opportunities for all riders from beginners to experts.

Map *Tahoe Rim Trail Map, Section 1*

Best Seasons Late June through November or up to the first major snow. After mild winters with less than average snow, it is possible to access this area by late May.

Highlights A gently rolling open forest makes for great riding on smooth trails. You will find beautiful meadows and several excellent lake views at the top of the climbs.

Heads Up! It's easy to get lost in the confusing trail pattern here. This is a busy area—watch out for hikers, dogs, children, horses, and bears.

Getting There From Tahoe City, take Highway 28 about 2.5 miles northeast to Fabian Way and turn left. Turn right on Village and proceed to the top of the hill, where Village veers right. Quickly turn left on Country Club Drive, and left again into the Tahoe Cross-Country Ski Area parking lot.

Brief Trail Description From the Nordic center, go up the dirt road heading west. This area has dozens of miles of trails that go to Tahoe City, Truckee, Northstar, or Brockway Summit. Mt. Watson is located at about 8 miles of steady climbing from the Nordic center where you'll have great lake views. Most trails are easy to moderate and very fun to ride. The opportunities for different rides are almost endless. For a detailed description of the Tahoe Rim Trail portion of this trail system, refer to the trail description for Section 1 (page 71).

Flume Trail and Tahoe Rim Trail Loop

Difficulty Strenuous 23-mile round-trip with a lot of climbing. The Flume Trail portion, which is 4.5 miles long, is on the edge of a cliff and may give the acrophobically challenged the heebie-jeebies.

Map *Tahoe Rim Trail Map, Section 3*

Best Seasons Mid-June through October

Highlights This is one of the most spectacular mountain biking routes in the United States. The views of Lake Tahoe are awe-inspiring, the fall colors can be extraordinary, and most of the trail is smooth and a treat to ride.

Heads Up! This very popular trail is used by both hikers and bikers and can be quite congested on weekends. Be especially cautious of hikers, and follow the posted bike speed limits. The 4.5-mile Flume Trail portion of the trail, while well constructed, may be challenging to those who fear heights.

Getting There The trailhead is off of Highway 28, about 0.5 mile from the intersection of Highways 28 and 50. It is located in Lake Tahoe Nevada State Park at Spooner Lake, about 27 miles from Tahoe City and 14 miles from South Lake Tahoe. A fee is required to park.

Brief Trail Description From the parking lot, head down a short hill to North Canyon Road, which you follow about 4 miles uphill to the saddle above Marlette Lake. There are maps at several kiosks along the route. A 1-mile descent takes you to a junction next to Marlette Lake. Turn left and follow the road around the west side of the lake to Marlette Lake's dam. To the left of the dam, the Flume Trail begins as a steep single track that quickly crosses the lake's outlet creek. For the next 4.5 miles the trail traverses, mostly level, over the location of the former water flume that ran from Marlette Lake to Carson City. This flume carried logs in the late 1800s to build Virginia City silver mines. The lake views from the Flume Trail are spectacular. Eventually the trail reaches Tunnel Creek Road.

If you would like a shorter ride, turn left and head down this road to Highway 28. In the summertime you can pay for a shuttle back to your car. Call (775) 749-5349 or go to **www.theflume trail.com** for shuttle information and times.

To continue on the Flume Trail and TRT loop, turn right and head up the steep hill 0.5 mile to the TRT, where you turn right. Follow the trail past Twin Lakes and begin climbing. The TRT heads mostly uphill for 2.4 miles and then mostly downhill for 2.7 miles to a junction at Hobart Road. Turn right on Hobart Road, and soon you will head downhill steeply to your junction next to Marlette Lake. Now you are retracing your route to the saddle above Marlette Lake and then on a long, fun downhill on North Canyon Road back to the trailhead.

Commemorative Emigrant Trail

Difficulty Easy to moderately difficult. For most people who have experience on single-track trails, this is a fun and not-too-difficult ride. It is a special treat for advanced riders looking for an opportunity to ride fast.

Best Seasons Late May to November. The snow on this trail usually melts earlier than that of any other single-track trail in the North Tahoe and Truckee area. After a mild winter you may be able to ride this trail by mid-April.

Highlights This is a fun ride with gentle ascents and descents through an open forest that strong riders can complete in about two hours. While the scattered forest scenery on this trail is pleasant, its great riding conditions are what make it especially enjoyable. Keep your eyes open for deer, which are commonly found along this trail.

Heads Up! Since in the spring this trail may be the only North Tahoe area mountain biking trail free of snow, it can be overcrowded, especially on weekends. As the snow melts and other trails become available, the number of riders on this trail drops significantly. In the middle of the summer this very exposed and dry trail can be quite hot and dusty.

Getting There Take Highway 89 about 4 miles north from the intersection of Interstate 80 and Highway 89 in Truckee. Just as you bridge Prosser Creek (the first large creek you pass heading north from Truckee), you will see a dirt parking area on the right side. Your trail starts here.

Brief Description The trail heads 9 miles north through a recently logged forest, eventually reaching Stampede Reservoir, where you turn around and return the same way. The trail intersects many dirt roads; just follow the well-labeled single-track trail. Along the route you see several meadows and Mt. Rose in the distance through the trees.

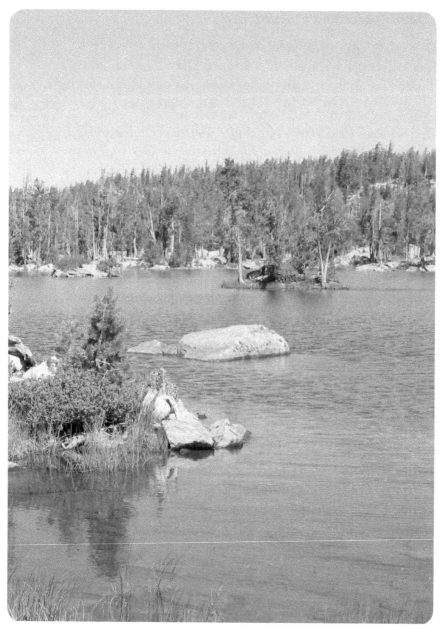

Middle Velma Lake

Afterword

Telling everyone about what the Tahoe Rim Trail has to offer is a joy to me. It is very satisfying to help others experience an incredible ridgetop view or the thrill of flying down a fun section of single-track trail. When I am guiding a trip and discussing the beauty around us, it is invigorating and restorative. That said, when I go out for a mountain bike ride on one of my favorite sections of trail, I get a bit irritated to see all those other people out there as well. Who are all these people, and why are they riding on this great trail that I used to have to myself? In writing this book, am I part of the problem? Am I fouling my own nest and the nest of others by telling everyone about the best places to go? Perhaps.

I hope that by providing the tools for people to enjoy their natural surroundings, I am increasing the understanding of how important it is for us to protect the natural world. If you enjoy this book and find it useful, please return the favor by doing what you can to protect what we still have and helping restore what has been damaged or destroyed. Go to work maintaining a trail. Join the Tahoe Rim Trail Association.

APPENDIX A

Resources and Amenities

Listed below are public agencies, Forest Service information centers, and other useful tidbits to help you plan your trip to the Tahoe Rim Trail.

National Forests

El Dorado National Forest
Information Center
3070 Camino Heights Drive
Camino, CA 95709
(530) 644-6048
www.r5.fs.fed.us/eldorado

Humboldt-Toiyabe National Forest
1536 South Carson Street
Carson City, NV 89701
(775) 882-2766
www.fs.fed.us/htnf

Lake Tahoe Basin Management Unit
35 College Drive
South Lake Tahoe, CA 96150
(530) 543-2600
www.fs.fed.us/r5/ltbmu

Tahoe National Forest
10342 Highway 89, North
Truckee, CA 96161
(530) 587-3558
www.r5.fs.fed.us/tahoe

Other Agencies

Lake Tahoe Nevada State Park
P.O. Box 8867
Incline Village, NV 89452
(775) 831-0494
www.state.nv.us/stparks/lt

Tahoe Rim Trail Association
DWR Community Non-Profit Center
948 Incline Way
Incline Village, NV 89451
(775) 298-0012
www.tahoerimtrail.org

Tom Harrison Maps
2 Falmouth Cove
San Rafael, CA 94901
(415) 456-7940
www.tomharrisonmaps.com

Useful Phone Numbers

Emergency: 911
Tahoe Nordic Search and Rescue: (530) 581-4038
El Dorado County sheriff: (530) 573-3000
Nevada County sheriff: (530) 582-7838
Placer County sheriff: (530) 581-6300
Washoe County sheriff: (775) 832-4107

Useful Websites

www.tahoerimtrail.org
Official website of the Tahoe Rim Trail Association.

www.writeonrex.com
Author's website about hiking, biking, mountain biking, cross-country skiing, and writing.

www.tahoetrips.com
Information about guided excursions at Lake Tahoe.

www.laketahoenews.com
Daily news headlines for Tahoe.

www.flyline.com
Information about fishing in the Sierra Nevada.

www.moonshineink.com
Truckee and Tahoe's great monthly news magazine.

www.tahoexc.org
Tahoe Cross-Country Ski Area website.

www.theflumetrail.com
Information about the Flume Trail shuttle.

www.kirkwood.com
Information about Kirkwood Downhill and Cross-Country ski areas.

www.tahoemtnmilers.org/trt50
Information about Tahoe Rim Trail endurance runs.

http://tahoe.usgs.gov
Your scientific portal to Lake Tahoe information.

APPENDIX B

Mileages for the Tahoe Rim Trail

The mileages for the distances between points along the Tahoe Rim Trail presented below are based on the cartographic work of the Tahoe Rim Trail Association, Jeffrey P. Schaffer, and Tom Harrison Maps.

Section Mileages (Clockwise)

Section Number	Location	Total Miles	Miles Between Points
Section 1	**Tahoe City to Brockway Summit**	**20.2**	
	Painted Rock		8.0
	Fiberboard Freeway Crossing		9.1
	Watson Lake		13.4
	Brockway Summit		20.2
Section 2	**Brockway Summit to Tahoe Meadows**	**20.2**	
	Spur Trail to viewpoint		1.2
	(viewpoint is 1.5)		
	Road to Martis Peak		4.3
	Rock Pile viewpoint		6.8
	Wilderness boundary		7.6
	Rose Knob Peak and Gray Lake junction		10.0
	Gray Lake junction and Mud Lake		11.2
	Relay Peak		14.6
	Wilderness boundary (dirt road)		15.0
	Via road (original TRT):		
	Mt. Rose Trail junction		16.4
	Mt. Rose Trailhead		19.6
	Via trail and Mt. Houghton Ridge:		
	Junction with Mt. Houghton Trail		15.5
	Junction with former TRT and		
	Snow Pond Trail		17.0
	Bottom of waterfall and Mt. Rose Summit		
	Trail junction		17.8
	Mt. Rose Trailhead		20.2

Section 8	Barker Pass to Tahoe City	16.7
	Twin Peaks Trail junction	4.8
	Twin Peaks on TRT	6.0
	Junction of TRT and	
	Stanford Rock Trail	6.3
	Ward Creek Road	11.5
	Tahoe City	16.7

Running Mileage (Clockwise)

Location	Clockwise Mileage	Mileage Between Points	Counter-clockwise Mileage
Tahoe City North Trailhead	0.0	20.2	173.2
Brockway Summit Trailhead	20.2	20.2	153.0
Mt. Rose Trailhead	40.4	0.8	132.8
Tahoe Meadows Trailhead	41.2	23.1	132.0
Spooner North Trailhead	64.3	—	108.9
Spooner South Trailhead	64.3	18.5	108.9
Kingsbury South Trailhead	82.8	23.2	90.4
Big Meadow Trailhead	106.0	15.3	67.2
Echo Summit Trailhead	121.3	2.2	51.9
Echo Lake Trailhead	123.5	32.7	49.7
Barker Pass Trailhead	156.2	16.7	17.0
Tahoe City South Trailhead	172.9	0.3	0.3
Tahoe City North Trailhead	173.2	—	0.0

Tim's Top 5 Places on the Trail

For Views

Dicks Pass (Section 7): Since it is quite a climb to reach the top of Dicks Pass, you'll want to spend some time enjoying the breathtaking views of two huge watersheds and a dozen lakes.

Christopher's Loop (Sections 3 and 4): Located about halfway between Tahoe Meadows and Spooner Summit at the end of a short spur trail, this viewpoint is not easy to reach, but you are rewarded with a view of of the entire lake and surrounding mountains (Section 3, page 112). The other great, east shore lake view is from South Camp Peak, halfway between Spooner Summit and Kingsbury Grade (Section 4, page 125).

Granite Chief Wilderness between Barker Pass and Twin Peaks (Section 8): Just south of the Pacific Crest Trail junction near Twin Peaks, at the end of a long climb, you reach a great open ridge, where you enter Granite Chief Wilderness. Views into the big valley of that wilderness and toward Desolation Wilderness and Lake Tahoe are spectacular. It's a perfect lunch spot.

Relay Peak (Section 2): The high point of this ridge in the Mt. Rose area is referred to as the "Million Dollar Mile" because it affords spectacular 360-degree views. On a clear day you can see the Sierra Buttes and Lassen Peak to your north.

Lake Aloha (Section 7): On a midsummer day without much wind, while you lounge on a rock with one foot in the water, gazing up at the Crystal Range is unbeatable.

To Swim

Lake Aloha (Section 7): Here is Lake Aloha again. What can I say? If you swim from island to island offshore when the water is warm, you will swear you have died and gone to heaven.

Middle Velma Lake (Section 7): This is another great lake for swimming, with numerous islands begging you to jump in and swim to them. If you are northbound on the TRT, it will be more than 80 miles before the next really good swimming lake (and that next lake is colder).

Truckee River and Lake Tahoe (intersection of Sections 1 and 8): Even though you cross the river right in the middle of Tahoe City, jump in and float around; it feels great. If you're ready for a break, consider a leisurely raft trip down the Truckee River; contact Mountain Air Sports at (530) 583-5606 for more information. Also the Commons Beach on Lake Tahoe in the center of Tahoe City is about 0.25 mile east of the Truckee River on Highway 28. If you are hiking the Tahoe Rim Trail, doesn't it make sense to swim in Lake Tahoe?

Star Lake (Section 5): Because of its high elevation, the lake can be extremely brisk (OK, it's bone-chilling cold), but the views are great and Star is the best lake along the east shore trail. If you hit it when it is warm, it makes for a great swim.

Showers Lake (Section 6): This lake has big, flat, granite rocks that go right down to the water's edge, which make for great swimming au naturel.

To Ride a Bike

Painted Rock (Section 1): Between Tahoe City and Brockway Summit, 2 miles in either direction of Painted Rock, is the smoothest, most enjoyable single-track trail you will ever ride. The easiest access point is Dollar Hill at the Tahoe Cross-Country Ski Area.

Tunnel Creek Road to Marlette Lake (Section 3): This portion of trail can be used as part of a loop with the Flume Trail. It includes some tough climbs and some thrilling downhills with spectacular views. Get off your bike to hike up to the view from Herlan Peak (aka Christopher's Loop).

Page Meadows (Section 8): The Page Meadows area, which has an extensive network of trails besides the Tahoe Rim Trail, offers some wonderful twists and turns on very ridable terrain. Stay out of the meadow itself until it dries up in the late summer or fall.

Spooner South to South Camp Peak (Section 4): This section offers great riding over sandy terrain with tremendous views along the way. Either turn around at the peak and enjoy the downhill stretch, or continue on to Kingsbury for something a little more challenging and technical.

Tahoe Meadows to Tunnel Creek (Section 3): Only available for use on "even" days of the month, this is probably the most popular mountain biking section on the TRT. After an initial climb, it is mostly downhill, with beautiful sandy conditions and great views. Some parts are pretty technical, but if you go on a summer weekend the most difficult challenge may be avoiding the crowds.

To Camp

Lake Aloha (Section 7): Hundreds of great spots are available on this big lake. It will give you privacy when the smaller Desolation Wilderness lakes are crowded.

Velma, Fontanillis, and Dicks Lakes (Section 7): All of these give you the full Desolation Wilderness experience, however crowded they become in midsummer. Very few campsites are available at Fontanillis.

Barker Pass (Section 8): About 2.5 miles north of Barker Pass is a peaceful little meadow with great views, a stream, and a nice camping spot among the trees.

Star Lake (Section 5): This lake is beautiful, the campsites have views of Tahoe as well as Star Lake, and the next lake is at least 17 miles away. Isn't it time to make camp? If you are feeling energetic, you can hike up to the top of Freel Peak in the morning; it's only 2 miles away.

Showers Lake (Section 6): Showers is a beautiful little lake offering great swimming and fine views. If you go there in the middle of the week, it might even be quiet and peaceful.

APPENDIX D

Ways to Save Lake Tahoe

We have been blessed with a deep blue alpine lake surrounded by majestic mountains. We must make an effort to preserve this lake and its environment so that future generations can enjoy it as well. The Tahoe Regional Planning Agency has come up with ways to save Lake Tahoe. A few of the best are listed below. These are a good place to start, but don't hesitate to think up your own.

1. **Take the bus. Share a ride. Take a hike. Ride a bike.** When you pick up your car keys, stop to plan the trip you're about to make. Can you run several errands while you're out? Could you save this trip until you need to make another? Is there another way you could get there? Reducing the number of trips you make and getting around without getting in your car reduces traffic congestion, helps protect air quality, and may improve your social skills and your health.

2. **Fill . . . don't spill.** If you fill it to the brim, gasoline may spill out of your tank and into Lake Tahoe.

3. **Skip a stone and leave the other rocks alone.** Rocks of all sizes and shapes are fish habitat. Fish need rocks to carry out their life cycles. Underwater rock gardens are where they spawn, feed, and hide from predators. By moving or rearranging rocks you might destroy valuable habitat.

4. **Don't be a trail blazer.** Erosion from unmaintained dirt roads presents a serious water-quality challenge. Off-highway vehicles and dirt bikes contribute to erosion when they travel off the maintained roads. Kids, stay on the designated roads. Parents, make sure your kids stay on the designated roads.

5. Take the beaten path. The tread from hiking boots and mountain bike tires are enough to cause erosion in the backcountry; it's best to stay on the trail.

6. You can lead a horse to water, but you shouldn't set up camp there. The less activity there is in a stream environment zone, the better. The law requires that you pitch your tent at least 200 feet from a body of water. That includes lakes, streams, creeks, reservoirs, and rivers.

7. Garbage in, garbage out. You could even pick up after a litterbug who went before you.

8. Finally, teach your children well.

The above information was provided as a courtesy of the Tahoe Regional Planning Agency. For more information, call them at (775) 588-4547.

Index

About the Author

Tim Hauserman has been a resident of North Lake Tahoe since 1960. He has hiked and biked in the area for many years and has been a guide for Tahoe Trips and Trails (a private excursion company), and the Tahoe Rim Trail. A member of the Tahoe Rim Trail

Board of Directors from 1998 to 2007, he became the 11th member of the Tahoe Rim Trail 165 Mile Club in 1999. His other books include *Monsters in the Woods: Backpacking with Children* and *Cross-Country Skiing in the Sierra Nevada.* He also writes for a variety of local and regional publications. Tim lives on the west shore of Lake Tahoe where he likes to hike, bike, cross-country ski, kayak, and practice yoga.